ADVANCE PRAISE
FOR *Finding Feminism*

An incredible, thought-provoking coming-of-age memoir studded with both painful and triumphant revelations. Overvoll is living proof that people can change, that experiences and relationships shape progress, and that questioning the status quo is crucial to growth.

—Niki Robins, Content Director, Spectacle Marketing

Finding Feminism is a captivating story of one woman's journey to connect with her true power—a story that I believe EVERY woman will be able to find herself in. I couldn't put it down!

—Lindsey Schwartz, Author of *Powerhouse Woman*

A beautifully written, emotionally provocative journey that will leave readers eager to kick the patriarchy's ass!

—Chelsea Duckham, COO of a Denver startup

Finding Feminism is captivating from cover to cover. Regardless of my own religious background, I felt as though this story was my own. It's raw, it's real, it's emotional. This book is a great read for anyone looking for how to grow and muster the strength it can take to move on.

—Kelly Kawa, Program Manager, Thinkful

As a woman, *Finding Feminism* hit close to home. It's beautifully written and tells the powerful story of Rachel taking back the power that the church, men, and her eating disorder had taken from her. The book brought tears to my eyes because my own personal experiences are so similar and because it shows the true strength of this woman. Rachel's memoir will leave you feeling empowered and in awe of the strength of all women.

—Julia Parzyck, FitFatAndAllThat and Eating Recovery Coach

Finding Feminism is an important story told boldly and tenderly through the voice of Rachel Overvoll who fought against an oppressive culture to find herself. Rachel's story is our story.

—Carly Gelsinger, Author of *Once You Go In*

Rachel Overvoll's memoir captivated me, making me feel like I was living right alongside her on her journey to break out of female oppression. Rachel's story will hit home no matter how liberated you think you are. An amazing story and a must read!

—Kelly Rice, Nutritionist

How delightful that a memoir exploring a seemingly extreme upbringing can powerfully convey universal struggles of womanhood. By immersing us in the insular world of purity balls, purity rings, and amiably rifle-holding fathers, Overvoll illuminates the larger ways in which our culture impacts each woman's sense of self. Overvoll's voice—vulnerable yet empowered—is intensely relatable. Readers will find comfort, courage, and insight in this story.

—Elizabeth Bailey, English Language Arts Curriculum Writer

Finding Feminism weaves together Rachel Overvoll's childhood memories of the Evangelical Christian community in which she was raised with the clear-eyed view of an adult who has a very different sense of what makes a good woman. Overvoll's love for her family and community is evident, but readers will recognize the pain and frustration she feels as she discovers a path markedly different from her family. Any woman examining her place in relationship to dating, sex, and partnership will learn from Overvoll's path to feminism.

—Sarah Woodard, English Language Arts Curriculum Developer

Rachel has spoken her truth in the most authentic, courageous, and vulnerable way. Her book is a captivating read. At points, I was totally engrossed in her God-centered world. As a champion for women, I can only hope that Rachel's book lands in the hands of those who need to read it the most.

—Edie Hortsman, Blogger of Wellness with Edie

finding *feminism*

a memoir

finding *feminism*

a memoir

Rachel Overvoll

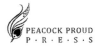

PEACOCK PROUD
P · R · E · S · S

PHOENIX, ARIZONA

Finding Feminism: A Memoir

First Published in the USA in 2019 by Peacock Proud Press, Phoenix, Arizona

ISBN 978-1-7322427-4-6 paperback
ISBN 978-1-7322427-5-3 eBook

Library of Congress Control Number: 2019938285

Editors:
Laura L. Bush, PhD, PeacockProud.com
Wendy Ledger, VoType.com

Cover and Interior Layout:
Melinda Tipton Martin, MartinPublishingServices.com

Portrait Photographer:
Carly M. Miller, Instagram.com/carlym.miller

DISCLAIMER:

This is a work of nonfiction. The information is of a general nature to help readers know and understand more about the life of the author, Rachel Overvoll. Readers of this publication agree that Rachel Overvoll, will not be held responsible or liable for damages that may be alleged or resulting directly or indirectly from their use of this publication. All external links are provided as a resource only and are not guaranteed to remain active for any length of time. The author cannot be held accountable for the information provided by, or actions resulting from accessing these resources.

To all the survivors
fighting for their voice and their power,
and to all the people who
helped me find mine.

#MeToo

Contents

THE LITTLE RED BOOK

My mom, a short woman with a red bob, metallic-framed glasses, and a constant smile, beamed as she walked into my room. "I have a surprise for you!" she sang.

She had just returned from Sherwood Baptist Church, the newly remodeled megachurch in Albany, Georgia, that my family attended. Our remodeled church included dozens of offices for the large pastoral staff, a two-story private prayer tower (open twenty-four hours a day in hopes that members of the church would be praying 24/7), a stage with room for an orchestra resembling a Broadway stage in New York City, and a brand new Christian bookstore.

Mom plopped down on my bed next to me and handed me a small red book with a pretty cursive font for its title, *Secret Keeper: The Delicate Power of Modesty*. Looking at me, she said, "I got this for you at the new bookstore at church. Rach, I think you're old enough to learn about the beautiful and Godly gift of purity." Then she smiled and kissed the top of my red wavy hair before leaving me alone with my new bright red book. The rest of the afternoon, I sat captivated, turning the ninety crisp pages while sitting on the bottom of the bunk bed I shared with my younger sister, Sarah.

We all know the age-old argument about whether a person is shaped by nature or nurture. I know both shaped me. My type A nature meant I grew up motivated, obsessed, and ambitious. Most likely, that's also why even as a child, all I ever wanted was to follow the rules to *perfection*. In my case, my family and the church nurtured me to obey the rules and to honor my family and my God. I believe my nature also gave me the desire to honor people deeply. Nurture, however, first led me to honor people according to the expectations of Evangelical Christianity. I wanted my family and my God to love me because I was good. In order to be "good," I had to follow the rules of Christianity, the rules of the Bible, the rules of the church, and, subsequently, the rules of my family. I had to follow all these rules to transcendence in order to be loved and admired.

From as young an age as I can remember, I heard my parents, grandparents, family, and church talk about the benefits of following the rules, of living a "God-fearing life." I wanted those benefits from God: *The blessings of eternal life. The blessings of joy. The blessings of a godly husband.* Following the rules and honoring God meant happiness and blessings. Dishonoring God meant spending eternity alone in Hell. Obviously, Heaven was the more attractive of the two options, so I sought God's will, truth, and approval. As a rule-follower, I deeply desired approval and was willing to do anything I was told to receive God's blessings, especially since the alternative to God's blessing was a scary pit of torture.

As I read that small red book on my bottom bunk bed in Albany, Georgia, I learned that modesty and abstinence would be two key factors for receiving God's blessings as I came into my womanhood. In other words, at only ten years old, the church began to teach me to view my worth in relation to my sexuality. According to this red book (and many sermons I would hear in the coming years), my value would be judged by how I expressed my sexuality. Reading page by page, I learned the role I needed to play as a "woman of God" and how I could best play this role. The author explained the necessity of dressing modestly in a "world filled with belly button rings and low-rise jeans."

"Wow!" I thought. "If I live my life without showing my body or giving it away before marriage, God will love me, and my parents will be proud of me. I will be good." That humid summer afternoon, I began to learn the value of myself in relation to modesty, abstinence, and the purity movement. What I didn't know, or even understand at the time, was that this small book would become the starting point for shaping my internal views about men, purity, my own body, and even feminism for the next twelve years.

CHILDHOOD

"The feminist agenda is not about equal rights for women. It is about a socialist, anti-family political movement that encourages women to leave their husbands, kill their children, practice witchcraft, destroy capitalism and become lesbians."

—Pat Robertson, 1992

The Altar and My Boobs

Religion, specifically Evangelical Christianity, was everything to my parents as they raised my sister and me. Both my mom and dad grew up in deeply religious, conservative households, and they transferred these passionately held beliefs to us while we were growing up. My dad worked at a government career that required us to move frequently, but moving to new towns and states never stopped my family from attending church services every Sunday morning, Sunday evening, and Wednesday night. My mother, a stay-at-home parent, spent her time homeschooling my sister and me while volunteering at our various churches. This led to us spending even *more* time within the institution of Evangelical Christianity. My mom found her source of community in the constructs of the church and, honestly, Sarah and I did too. My mom didn't have a normal, ongoing community of work friends. Since Sarah and I were homeschooled, we had to find our friends at church. In fact, we spent at least four days a week at the church. According to my parents, the church provided all answers and the absolute truth. It offered them community and provided a sanctuary for religious devotion. Because of what the church meant to my parents, it became my set of regulations, too.

My dad's job stationed us in Albany, Georgia, about one month before my eighth birthday. We were stationed there for four years while he worked forty minutes north in Plains, Georgia, protecting former President Jimmy Carter. When we moved to a new city, my family always church shopped for a few weeks. We would visit a specific church for the Sunday morning service, then Mom and Dad would pray all afternoon. In their prayers, they asked God if we should attend the Sunday evening service at the same church. If God laid it on my parent's hearts to attend the Sunday evening service, then they would pray all week until they felt God told them to either a) keep shopping or b) become a member of that church. A few Sundays after our move, at the end of their Sunday afternoon prayers, Mom and Dad had decided that God wanted us to attend Sherwood Baptist Church, a megachurch with more than 2,000 attendees every Sunday. The church was grandiose, and my parents said the sermons were "filled with the fire of the Lord."

On Sunday morning, church service lasted for two hours, and

there was another hour-long service in the evening. The church held what felt like, to a young girl, 10,000 people and smelled like fresh paint because it had recently been remodeled. As a young girl, I felt completely overwhelmed by the large dark stage, the full orchestra, the 100-member choir, and the two levels of stadium seating. To me, God felt infinitely large in this larger-than-life building. We began every Sunday service with praise and worship music, then moved on to a message by our pastor, who jokingly said on many occasions, "I look like a marshmallow with two toothpicks for legs!" (It's true; he did.)

After the marshmallow pastor finished his sermon, we bowed our heads to pray. When we opened our eyes after the prayer, the worship team, orchestra, and choir would be ready to perform on the stage—like a magic trick. The worship leader, Mac, then extended the invitation to come to the altar as they began playing an assortment of praise and worship music, always centered around the theme that we are sinners and unworthy of everything God has done for us. *God is everything. I am nothing.* The dim lights raising back to life, as the 100-member choir began singing. The belief was that, if you came to the pews in the front of this overwhelming large arena, other members of the congregation could see you and pray for you from the comfort of their darkened seat. In concept, the ceremony seems genuine and wholesome. In reality, it became the church's favorite channel for gossip. I remember hearing my parents and their friends wonder why someone, "has gone to the altar a lot in the last month, bless their heart. Do you know what's going on?"

I remember going down to the altars that lined the front of the church stage almost every Sunday morning and night to cry and repent for my "sins." My Sunday School teachers taught me all about sins—a long list of actions including gossip, being mean to your parents or siblings, cursing, not reading your Bible, or not telling at least one "unsaved" soul about God every day (evangelizing). As I entered the youth group in sixth grade, the teachers added more sins to the list, including dressing immodestly, looking at men with lust, flirting, sex outside of marriage, dating without God's blessing, and dating a non-Christian.

I went to the altar frequently because the thought of being unholy terrified me.

Sherwood Baptist taught me that, if I died at any minute but had not repented from a sin that I committed a mere minute before, I would end up in hell, thanks to my most recent unconfessed transgression. That church taught me about a lot of sins, so I had a lot to fear. Looking back, I believe my terror resulted from high anxiety combined with the church's teachings. In case you're wondering, in the evangelical community, anxiety is similarly viewed as depression and is another "sin," one I often asked to be forgiven for during those front-and-center occasions. My youth leaders also taught me about these sins. They explained, "For heavy worry or heavy sadness to occur in your life, you must not be living in God's will or trusting God with everything you have. If you live with total trust in the Lord, you will live a joy-filled, worry-free life." I bought it completely.

Church elders and my parents always expressed how proud they were of me for my bravery and honesty in tackling my sins. My frequent walk to the front of the church altar was not only lauded, but also encouraged by the adults in my life, even though they must have known that I would be gossiped about after the ritual. Was this something so ingrained in our culture that we didn't realize the harm of the ritual? That the idea of encouraging a child to feel shame and thus repent publicly may be more detrimental than holy? At that time and at my young age, I only viewed my altar prayers as holy, which felt validated by my parents' praise and support.

Going through puberty at the megachurch, I began to frequent the altar not for gossiping or being mean to my sister, but because I felt guilty about the way my body was changing. One Sunday morning, my mom and I were in the church parking lot waiting for the attendees to flag us through the busy traffic with a walk sign. My normally effervescent mom looked forward with hesitation in both her voice and her face, as she said, "Honey, I need to talk to you as soon as we get home . . . then we can make lunch together." At the time, I didn't think anything of what she said, but when we got home, she immediately swept me into my bedroom for privacy and sat down with me on my bottom bunk.

I loved that magical bedroom decorated with lime green, electric blue, and bright yellow flowers. Even as the older sister, I slept on the bottom bunk, my safe place because heights have always alarmed me. I refused to sleep on or even climb up to the top bunk of the bed. Except for this one time. One evening, my dad had insisted that I climb up to Sarah's top bunk before bedtime to make me "overcome my fears." Sitting on that top bunk, anxiety filled my entire being. I hyperventilated and sobbed. He had to pick me up and put me on the floor because I was so paralyzed by the fear. Sitting here on my bottom bunk, waiting to hear what my mom wanted to tell me, I felt secure.

"Rachel . . . " she said, sitting next to me, "I think it's time for you to get a bra."

"Why?" I asked, confused. In my mind, my body was normal, and in all honesty, I loved the way my breasts felt when they were free against my T-shirt, unbound by some contraption I knew I would have to wear for the rest of my life.

My mom was a flute player in the church orchestra and had overheard a conversation. She sighed. "Some of the women in the choir were talking, and they said your breasts are too big and are causing a distraction for their sons at church. They . . . um . . . asked me to get you a bra." She spoke these words with delicacy, heavy with shame on my behalf. There on my bed, at the age of ten, was the first moment I became painfully aware of my body. My body, in its naked state, felt disgraceful. I felt angry and helpless because I had no control over this new development. My breasts had just appeared, and now I had to rein them in? It seemed unfair.

We went to Wal-Mart to buy a bra before the church service that night—a pure white unlined training bra with a small pink bow in between my breasts. I wore this under my baggy white T-shirt in an effort to hide my body in its entirety. After the choir sang and the pastor with the toothpick legs and marshmallow body preached, I went to the front of the big dark church to pray at the altar again. This time, though, my transgression had changed. I asked God to forgive me for my deceitful body.

Cotillion

In sixth grade, all my friends from church signed up for Cotillion, an eight-week course teaching etiquette and basic ballroom dance. In reality, it was more a course on status, where the wealthy sent their children to be more like them, and where the middle-class families would scrape together every extra cent they made to send their children to the upper echelon.

We were never the richest family, but we weren't poor by any means either. We were firmly middle-class. A few years before my dad was born, his parents emigrated from Norway to realize the American Dream. Both of my paternal grandparents survived the Nazi occupation of Norway. Neither of them had received an education past the eighth grade. They were wonderful grandparents and worked very hard to provide my father with what they had lacked in their own childhoods. They passed on this generosity to my dad, who tried to do the same for my sister and me.

My mom came from a small farming community in upstate New York. The town is so small that, to this day, I receive no cellphone service when visiting my grandfather's farm. As a daughter of dairy farmers and a son of immigrants, my parents had worked hard and attained the coveted American middle-class status. Obviously, Cotillion wasn't cheap. My parents were incredibly proud that they had saved all of my dad's extra earnings to send me to such a prestigious club. They had made it, and their daughter could now make it farther.

Every week for the first seven weeks of Cotillion, we learned table etiquette and simple ballroom dance steps. The classes were held in a ballroom in an upscale country club, way beyond the means of my parents. Every week they would drop me off with such joyful satisfaction as they chatted and waved to the parents who were actually members of the club. The club entryway was covered in light pink carpet that welcomed you into a large ballroom with scuffed wooden floors (from dancing) and dark maroon curtains. It smelled like stale cigar smoke, freshly mown grass from the greens outside, and stale cologne from the boys who had borrowed their fathers' bottles before coming to class. About a dozen round tables surrounded the dance floor. We sat decorously at them to practice our table manners, before heading to the dance floor for our ballroom dance lessons. On Sunday afternoons between our morning and evening church services, we met for two hours in this odd and elegant country club.

During our two-hour Sunday meetings, the leaders of Cotillion enforced a strict dress code. For our classes, the girls were required to wear a skirt or dress while boys had to wear slacks and a button-down shirt with a tie. Bob and Jean, the married couple who led our classes, organized, arranged, and perfectly instructed everything in our aristocratic bubble. They did this in preparation for the final class—The Ball. This would be our one and only test during the eight weeks of discipline to become true ladies and gentlemen. It would be an evening for ten- to twelve-year-olds to dress in gowns and suits, eat a formal dinner with our finest table manners, and demonstrate our basic ballroom dance knowledge.

When the night of The Ball arrived, I could not contain my giddy excitement. For the last eight weeks, I had daydreamed about this Cinderella night. It was finally here! I wore a hot pink strapless, sparkly dress, cut in an A-line. My mom and I had glee-fully found it at Dillard's in the after-prom sale section for $20, which luckily fit our dress budget. I paired it with long white gloves and two-inch black heels. I wrapped the hot pink dress in a graceful black silk shawl that my Norwegian grandmother, Nana, had sewed for me especially for the event. My parents had only agreed to purchase the hot pink strapless gown for me if I promised to wear the black silk shawl all night to cover my shoulders. The new $20 dress did not leave a lot of extra money in our ball budget so Nana, being the seamstress that she was, sewed a shawl perfectly suited for my new pink dress. About two weeks before Cotillion, Nana and I had gone to Wal-Mart together to look through the limited amount of fabric they sold in order to find the perfect material for the shawl. She always said, "If it's more than $5, then it's not worth it." So, of course, we found our fabric at the local Wal-Mart. I didn't mind wearing the shawl. In fact, I loved how I felt when I wrapped it around my shoulders. I knew that, without the shawl, the dress might cause men to sin. I didn't want God to hold me responsible for that action, so I covered my shoulders to preserve my innocence. The little red book about modesty continued to have an impact on me.

Mom had paid to have my hair styled, and I wore a glamorous low bun in my hair with loose curls falling around my face. A small amount of Queen Anne's lace was woven into the delicate bun. My parents did everything they could to make this a magical night for me. I felt absolutely beautiful.

I arrived at the country club around 6:00 p.m., and my parents took pictures with me before quickly saying their goodbyes, so I could begin my showcase night. We had dinner first, where we were all placed at eight-person tables with equal boy-girl ratios. Since our entire class was made up of mostly girls, our instructors, Bob and Jean, had recruited their son and some of his friends, who had completed the middle-school Cotillion course, to sit at our tables to fill in any gaps for the dance numbers. In addition to Bob and Jean grading our every movement, the older boys had volunteered to not only eat and dance with the young class, but to grade our formalities as well.

After the five-course dinner, the dancing began. Most sixth graders are very awkward. I was no exception. Despite the visit to the salon, the Georgia humidity had turned my curly locks into a frizzy mess. Smiling revealed my braces. My 4'9" frame housed my 32C chest and a large butt. I was the epitome of early blooming with no idea of how to handle any of it. When the dancing began, I stood against the wall on the side of the country club ballroom, hoping that a boy would ask me to dance. I watched as, girl by girl, everyone was asked to dance while I stood alone, waiting in anticipation. The first dance began. It was a waltz, but still no one had asked me to dance. Bob and Jean's son stepped in. He asked me to dance out of obligation, knowing his role for the evening. Although I understood his responsibility at this event, his manners and kind smile made me feel less unwanted as we moved across the dance floor.

The second song played, and again no one asked me to dance. So a different older boy asked me to dance. I instantly recognized him as a friend of Bob and Jean's son. We chatted and laughed as we danced a quick fox-trot. He seemed friendly. I felt important dancing with him. He was almost three years older than me! In the way he spoke to me and looked at me, I felt noticed for the first time that evening. Even as I tried to remind myself of his obligation at this event, he made me feel chosen. The next song started, and again I was standing alone waiting for someone to ask me to dance. When the song began and I leaned against the wall on the outskirts of the dance floor, the same cute older boy approached and asked me to dance. With my metal-filled smile, I beamed as he took my hand and guided me to the dance floor.

We were attempting a cha-cha when I felt his hand slide down my lower back. *Okay, I thought. It's only my lower back.* But slowly his hand kept sliding downward until he firmly planted it on my butt. I assumed that it was an accident. When the song ended, I moved to the side of the floor to wait for a new suitor to ask me to dance for the next song. I ended up being solo again, so the cute older boy asked me to dance for the third time. This time we danced a waltz. His hand again moved to my butt and, this time, he pinched it. I froze, shocked. Several more times throughout the night I stood alone as the songs began, and he continued to ask me to "dance." He would wait until my back was turned to a wall so no one could see his lingering hand. With each song, realizing I wouldn't protest, he became emboldened. He groped and pinched me repeatedly. Fear filled my eleven-year-old mind, causing my body to freeze and move robotically through the dances I had worked so hard to perfect.

After my parents picked me up that night, my mom helped

me remove dozens of bobby pins from my hair and wash off my lipstick. I put on my dad's XL Secret Service T-shirt, which I frequently wore to bed, and I lay silently in my bottom bunk. I remember thinking to myself, "This didn't happen. I must have imagined it. How could a handsome Cotillion gentleman do this? He couldn't have because he learned to be a gentleman. I must have made it up in my head."

I went to sleep with this argument raging inside my head. *Was this real? Did this actually happen to me? Was I going crazy? Can an eleven-year-old go crazy?* I woke up in the middle of the night, crying uncontrollably. Sarah woke up from her top bunk, crawled down into my bed, and tried to settle me down. She stroked my hair and curled herself around my shaking body, but when she realized that I could not be consoled, she ran to my parents' bedroom across the house and woke up my mom. Mom came into our room instantly, knelt on the side of my bed, and tenderly wiped my tears from my red face as she asked what was wrong. I didn't respond to her questions because I didn't know or understand what was wrong. I thought I might have gone crazy. I cried and cried, but I knew no words to express what had happened to me that evening—sexual assault. He had taken advantage of me, and I didn't have the words to understand what had happened. After Mom and Sarah comforted me for a while, I finally muttered, "He grabbed me over and over again."

"Who grabbed you over and over again, baby?" my mom

asked softly, with the tenderness only a mother has for her child.

Tears continued to roll down my face as I choked out, "The boy who I danced with all night."

Mom and Sarah laid with me in the twin bunk bed until my body calmed down enough to fall asleep.

The following morning, my parents called Bob and Jean so they could discuss what had happened to me the night before. To our collective surprise, the boy who had assaulted me was not only the best friend of their son, but he was also the son of *their* best friends. I remember sitting in our living room, hiding so I could listen to my parents' hushed voices through the wall to the kitchen, discussing the incident over the phone with Bob and Jean. My dad, with all his negotiation training, took the lead on the call.

"Rachel was very upset last night . . ."

"She . . . um . . . said that that boy kept grabbing her butt all night."

"So, no one saw this?"

"How do you normally handle these situations?"

"Oh . . . so this has never happened before?"

"Yes, I think a group meeting with everyone would be good. We can talk through what happened and hear both kids. We understand this is upsetting for everyone."

Later that week, we had a group meeting with him, his family, Bob, Jean, my parents, and me. To my naïve amazement, the boy denied everything and his parents backed him up. I knew what had happened that night and what he had taken from me, so it astonished my young mind that a boy would lie to all of us regarding what he had done to my body. He not only lied, but his parents and Bob and Jean were eager to believe him. They spoke their truth, then we spoke ours.

There came a point in the evening when everyone realized that this situation could not be resolved since neither parents would budge on their unwavering advocacy for their children. When this moment arrived, Bob, Jean, and his parents agreed that it would be best if I did not continue the Cotillion courses. The boy would continue to be a leader for the younger students, but I could no longer attend the classes in order to "reduce any tensions." My parents were not pleased with the resolution, but they also wanted an end to this incident. Parents don't want to focus on an injustice someone has committed against their child. My parents have always been especially good at sweeping the uncomfortable moments in life under the rug.

Driving home from the meeting that evening, my dad said, "God will test you, honey. I am glad you stood up for yourself and stood strong. You must rely on the purpose God has for you in all of this." *God has a plan.* This would be the only time my parents ever spoke of this incident again.

This would also be the first time, but certainly not the last, that I realized that some people are eager to believe boys and men "could never do something like that" before they will ever consider that a girl or a woman is telling the truth about being assaulted.

The Pure White Ball

In seventh grade, my family moved across the state from Albany to St. Simons Island, Georgia, a small island connected to the mainland by a 4.2-mile causeway covering a large marsh. It reeked of the smells of stagnant water and decaying plant material, a nauseating odor of sulfur and rotten eggs. Given the stench surrounding it, I often thought it odd that St. Simons Island was a vacation destination; its economy relied on tourism, and summer visitors made the island vibrant with energy. I remember almost vomiting the first time my family drove over the causeway.

On that hot July day, my mom rolled down the windows on our white Ford minivan—unaware of the new odor welcoming us to our small island home. I think the combination of the marsh entryway and my anxiety of starting all over again in a new town caused my queasiness. Since, as a Christian, I wasn't supposed to feel anxious, I told my mom the stench of the island caused my nausea, purposely leaving out my all-consuming and "sinful" anxiety.

We had to move because my dad had been promoted—he was now an instructor at the Federal Law Enforcement Training Center (FLETC), a step forward for his career with a much less demanding schedule. My dad was thrilled. In Albany, he had to work strange hours while protecting former President Carter. Now he could spend more time with his family and go out on his much-loved fishing expeditions. However, Sarah and I were hardly delighted. We would have to leave all of our megachurch friends behind, and Mom and Dad still planned to homeschool us. As we grew older, we found it more and more challenging to make friends outside of a traditional school setting. Moving and continuing our education at home forced us to again make friends within a church of my parents' choosing.

With the move, we church shopped again. Every Sunday we attended a new church. After the service, my parents would pray together and wait to feel God's presence telling them if they should become members of that church or keep shopping. After visiting about five different churches, my parents finally found one that they believe God wanted them to attend. The new church was much smaller than the megachurch, and services were held in the second-story business front of a strip mall. I felt relieved when they picked this church as our home base. Finding a church meant I no longer had to place a pause on my social life. I could now make friends at this new church where my parents had decided to stay.

At my first Wednesday youth group meeting, my youth pastor, Hannah, stepped onto the stage to make the closing announcements. The worship music had just ended in the small dark room in the shopping center. I sat next to Sarah as Hannah announced a collaborative church event happening the following month: The Purity Ball. Hannah, a tall blonde with glowing tan skin from too many afternoons at the beach, coyly described the event. "This is a women's only event," she said. "And I would like to discuss the details with you personally. Please come see me after youth group if you'd like more info." Then she led us in a closing prayer. After the prayer, I looked at Sarah and asked, "Want to go?"

"If it means we get to dress up!" she said enthusiastically.

Desperate to make new friends, we both found Hannah after the meeting and asked her for more information about the event.

"So, what do we need to do to go?" we asked her.

Hannah replied with an ecstatic smile. "Fill out this form, and make sure your dad can escort you. He'll need to bring rings to give you girls for the ceremony, but that's all you need to do after you register!"

"Cool!" Sarah and I said in unison. Then Sarah, who was still too young to have attended the Cotillion classes or ball, added, "We get to dress up and dance, right?"

"Of course!" replied Hannah. "I am so proud that you're taking this step toward purity. Pledging your body to God before marriage is such a special commitment—and totally even more special when your dad pledges with you."

"Sweet!" Sarah responded as she high-fived Hannah.

We were in and sure to make some new friends at the ball! Our dad picked us up from the youth group that evening in our family minivan. As soon as we climbed into the van, we excitedly told him about the event and asked if he would escort us. Beaming as he accelerated through a green light, he replied, "Of course! I'm so glad you want to go to this — I think it's really sweet! Stuff like this is why I took my new job. It's so great to be off on evenings to spend time with my girls." When we got home, he filled out the registration forms. Then he took us ring shopping later that week, so we could each pick out our perfect purity ring. I picked out a small silver band, and Sarah decided on a small gold band, both simple and classic.

For the Purity Ball, I reused my hot pink dress from Cotillion. Sarah got to go shopping for a new dress because she had never been to a formal event. I begged my mom for a new dress the day she took Sarah shopping (again in the 75 percent off prom dress section of Dillard's), but as she moved her hands through the racks of dresses, she insisted, "Your Cotillion dress looks lovely on you, and you've only worn it once! You don't need to be wasteful." But I wanted to move on from what had happened at Cotillion a few months before. Something in me kept saying a new dress at a new ball would help me forget the boy who had groped me and the adults who hadn't believed me. However, my frugal mom stuck to her decision. I needed to push the incident out of my mind and wear the pink dress. *God has a plan.*

The night of the ball, I was eager to meet new friends, and

I looked forward to the ceremony. This simple pledge would honor God and make my parents proud of me. After tonight, any shame my body had brought to my parents or to God from the last time I had worn this dress would disappear. Everyone would see my public dedication to God and be proud of me. *God has a plan.* Sarah's excitement, on the other hand, came from her new dress and the opportunity to dance the night away. We put on our dresses, mine pink with the black shawl Nana had sewn, and Sarah's floor-length, bright blue metallic dress with spaghetti straps. Mom tried to curl and pin our hair on her own, in order to save a costly trip to the salon. Everything on an island is more expensive, even the salons. Since I have naturally curly hair while my sister and mom have naturally straight hair, Mom's attempts at styling my hair never ended up going well. After neatly pinning up Sarah's straight, thin hair and spending about thirty minutes trying to tame my curls, Mom finally said with frustration, "Well, Rach. I don't know what to do here." She really wanted to make it nice, and my Medusa curls made her feel like a failure. I convinced her that I would love to wear my hair down with its natural curls. At least my hairstyle would be different from the last time I had to wear this dress.

We arrived right on time that night, a rarity for my parents and Sarah, who always run at least thirty minutes behind schedule. My eagerness swiftly propelled everyone out the door of our small island house. Tonight, we would *not* be late! Dad, with his cleanly shaven bald head and all-black suit, rolled up to the entry-way in our minivan to drop us off before parking the car. This is something he will still do to this day with all of the women in his family, even as he closes in on his sixties. He likes to drop off the "ladies at the entrance because it is the gentlemanly thing to do." After he parked the car, he met us at the entrance to escort us arm in arm into the ball. As soon as I entered the large event room, the brightness of everything struck me. Everything was white: the paint on the walls, the tablecloths, the chairs, the banners with the emblem, all the desserts. They had even brought in large white runners to cover up the majority of the light wooden dance floor. The large ballroom, with about 200 daughters and their fathers in attendance, beamed white like a sterile hospital room. When we entered, a young woman in a light-yellow dress asked our names before escorting us to our table. Another father-and-daughter duo had already sat down at our shared dining area. The father stood and shook Dad's hand, introducing himself as Hank before introducing his stepdaughter Jen. Hank wore an ill-fitting gray suit with a light-yellow collared shirt, and Jen wore a simple floor-length black gown. She was one year younger than me and one year older than Sarah, so we quickly began gabbing together. As Sarah, Jen, and I sat at the table and talked about how dreamy Aaron Carter was, the merits of the Backstreet Boys vs. N'Sync, riding our bikes to the beach, and painting our nails, Dad and Hank were reverently discussing the importance of this event.

I remember overhearing Hank say to my dad, "I'm trying to be a good father figure, ya know? I think bringing Jen here shows that . . . or I hope it does."

In Dad's Brooklyn accent, he applauded Hank, "Yes! It absolutely does. I think this is a really beautiful event. Those boys out there are going to try to use our baby girls, and we have to protect them."

Shortly after we sat down, ethereal elevator music began, commencing the event. A petite balding man with wire-rimmed glasses took the podium in the center of the white ballroom. An ornamental white cross framed the space behind him. He began the evening with the typical verbose gratitude any emcee uses to speak to the guests of an event. Then he reached under the podium to bring out a beautifully packaged present: a square box, wrapped in pearly, shimmering wrapping paper with a silver bow draped around it. We all sat, silently waiting for the petite man to explain the purpose behind the present. He began the program, "Can I have five male volunteers come up here?" Five men, including Dad, stood up and walked to meet the emcee in the center of the room. The emcee continued, "I would like for you volunteers to pass this present down the line. As you pass it to the man next to you, rip a piece of the wrapping off." One by one, the fathers passed the present down the line as they ripped it apart. After the package ended at the last father in the line, the emcee asked him, "How do you feel about this present? Do you want it?" The father quickly replied, "No! It looks mangled." The emcee looked at the room. "You see, ladies," he explained as he walked between the round white tables, orating like a poor man's Tony Robbins, "This present is an example of your purity. It is a gift meant for one man and one man *only*. Do you think the man God has chosen for you will want to open a mangled gift that was meant for him but has been torn apart by other men?"

Listening to the emcee, I was enthralled. It all made so much sense. I needed to be pure, not only for God and for my family, but also so that my future husband, who God has already appointed, actually wants me. If I'm damaged, he won't want me! *The blessings of a godly husband.* Interrupting my thoughts, Sarah leaned over and whispered into my ear, "This is kinda weird. Do you think the dancing will start soon?"

"SHHHH!!!" I shot back. I wanted to hear everything the emcee was saying, so I knew how to get a godly husband.

The emcee then asked the volunteers to return to their tables to recite the purity pledge to their daughters. The pledge was printed on a card placed in the center of our table. The emcee instructed our fathers to read aloud in unison: "I, (daughter's name)'s father, choose before God to cover my daughter as her authority and protection in the area of purity. I will be pure in my own life as a man, husband, and father. I will be a man of integrity and accountability as I lead, guide, and pray over my daughter and my family as the high priest in my home. This covering will be used by God to influence generations to come."

Sarah and I stood as Dad read the pledge to us. Then he slipped our new rings on each of our wedding fingers—my silver band with a small cubic zirconia in the middle and Sarah's gold band with the cubic zirconia. The rings were significant, the first adult pieces of jewelry either of us had ever owned, and now an ever-present reminder of our virginity pledge to both Dad and God. The emcee instructed us to wear our rings daily until we received a wedding ring from the man God had prepared for us.

After his instructions, he led us in a prayer for purity that included requests such as, "God save these women from the young men who will try to steal their soul," or "God make these women strong and remember that you are their groom until they meet the man you have ordained for them," and "God help these women to dress in a way that does not cause any men of Christ to stumble into sin." We all said "amen" in unison, and then the dance floor opened with Bob Carlisle's "Butterfly Kisses."

Sarah immediately looked at Dad with her big bright blue eyes and said, "FINALLY dancing! Can we dance?" My dad grabbed her hand and led her to the dance floor. I sat at the table, listening to "Butterfly Kisses," watching my dad spin Sarah as they danced in that white room, feeling so proud of myself. "I am a good young woman, a godly woman." I thought. I felt honored to make both my earthly and heavenly father proud of me. I felt secure that making this purity promise would provide me a godly husband. *God's Blessings.* My virginity made me a rare, deeply desired prize. Any godly man will crave me now. *My value is virginity. Sex outside of marriage will leave me abandoned.*

HIGH SCHOOL AND ENGAGEMENT

"True love isn't just expressed in passionately whispered words or an intimate kiss or an embrace; before two people are married, love is expressed in self-control."

—Joshua Harris, *I Kissed Dating Goodbye: A New Attitude Toward Relationships and Romance*

Saved

The summer before ninth grade, my family moved to northwest Indiana. We traded in the warm Georgia beach for gray skies above and steel mills below, but once again, Dad's job had brought us here. Portage is about forty-five minutes outside of Chicago, so although the population is less than forty thousand, at least we were close to the metropolitan Windy City. Dad had taken a promotion in Chicago, requiring him to commute across the Indiana border daily to the Secret Service office there.

Mom and Dad had chosen to live in Portage over Chicago because Portage is halfway between my grandparents' house in South Bend, Indiana, and Dad's office in Chicago. Despite the dreary weather and dismal small-town appearance, Sarah and I found an upside, an adventure, to this move. Mom and Dad promised us this would be our last move as a family, guaranteeing Sarah and me that we would complete high school in the same town. My parents had chosen to homeschool us up until this point because they believed it provided greater consistency as we moved from different towns and states. Now that we were stationary for my final four years of high school, Mom and Dad thought it would be best for Sarah and me to enter a traditional school setting. No more moves. No more isolated homeschooling. We could now create an actual foundation for our lives without worrying when our existence would be uprooted again.

Although my parents had decided that we would enter a traditional education setting, they had only considered private Christian education. Public school, as they said, "promotes liberal ideas, is where kids lose their faith in God, and doesn't keep kids safe." When they told us the public school horror stories that they heard on Fox News or through their "Growing Kids God's Way" monthly emails, I'm not sure if they meant to scare us, or if they'd actually believed the stories they were told. Either way, Sarah and I were also convinced that private Christian school safeguarded us from the evils of the outside world. Because Portage is such a small town, the options for a private Christian education were limited to one school: Portage Christian School or PCS, a small PK-12 school about seven minutes away from our house, with a stated mission of "Imparting God's Wisdom for Godly Living through the Educational Process."

I can still vividly picture that first day of school. I spent all morning in my bathroom at home, meticulously straightening my red hair until all my natural curls had disappeared. Then I put on the little makeup I had purchased from Wal-Mart with my babysitting money—CoverGirl black eyeliner and a light pink shimmery blush. I chose to wear a blue polo shirt with dark blue jeans that I had found in the sale section at our local mall. I looked in the mirror with confidence—ready to begin my next chapter with new friends and adventures. I had thirsted for this experience for so long. Portage Christian School would offer me a daily community of Christian friends and the academic challenges I had been craving.

Mom, who is late for almost everything, surprisingly dropped Sarah and I off twenty minutes before the first bell rang on that humid August morning. Pulling up to the drop-off lane, she asked us to bow our heads and close our eyes for a quick prayer. "God, please bless Sarah and Rachel today as they enter a new school. Please provide friends for them and protect them from evil. Amen." With that, we jumped out of the minivan and walked into our new school.

That morning, Sarah had opted for turquoise eye shadow all over her eyelids, matching her electric blue skirt. She's always been the bold one and walked in front of me, so she was the first to be greeted by our new principal, Mr. Rumble. He was tall, over six feet, with large lips, and long, slicked back hair, so thin that you could see his scalp. Introducing himself in a reserved fashion to Sarah first, then me, he welcomed us to our new school and asked that we make our way to the chapel for a sermon to start our day.

There were two hallways in that school, one off the entryway that led right to all the PK-grade five classrooms, and the other, which led left to the classrooms for middle school and high school students as well as the chapel. I looked down at the carpet—an old navy blue with stains so deep that from afar you might mistake them for a pattern. The walls were tan, lined with yellow metal lockers. With my polka dot backpack held close to me, I made my way down the secondary hallway to the chapel room. Sarah and I sat next to each other as we watched other students slowly trickle in. No one said anything to us or even noticed us. As I watched the friend groups forming around me, my anxiety began to rise, and my excitement began to fade as I realized that I didn't belong in any of these groups. The room suddenly felt alienating.

After about twenty minutes of my anxious thoughts running rampant through my mind, Mr. Rumble walked to the front of the chapel room and greeted us. He started the morning with a prayer, then moved into addressing the handbook. His large lips pursed and spit as he went rule by rule through the school handbook: "P.D.A.: Students are not allowed to show inappropriate Public Displays of Affection. These include but are not necessarily limited to: Kissing." A group of boys near me chuckled. Mr. Rumble paused his oration, staring at the group of boys with severity. They immediately stopped their snickers and looked down. As Mr. Rumble continued, I learned that holding hands, full frontal hugging of the opposite gender, sitting on the lap of the opposite gender, riding on the back of the opposite gender, and touching the leg of the opposite gender were all also "inappropriate in the eyes of God" and not allowed.

Considering that no one had even noticed me enough to say hello, I didn't think these rules would be a problem for me this year. He read each rule with a corresponding Bible verse to make us all aware of exactly where God had called us to these standards. I listened intently to each rule, so I knew exactly how to present myself. If anyone broke the rules, detention or expulsion would be mandated, depending on the severity of the rule breaking. Mr. Rumble made that very clear.

After the welcome meeting in the chapel, we all made our way to our own classrooms. Class by class, my new teachers asked me to walk to the front of the room to introduce myself. Through this awkward exercise, I quickly realized that all my classmates had gone to school here together since they were in elementary school. In the entirety of the ninth-grade class, I was the only new girl. Everyone here had deep roots and connections. I was the outsider.

Day after day for the next several months, I would go to school filled with hope but leave feeling so alone. All summer I had envisioned walking into PCS and being met with kindness from the other students. In my naivety, I thought that as soon as I entered those doors, a group of girls would invite me to eat lunch with them, and we would all quickly begin sharing secrets and lip gloss. But this was high school. Teenagers aren't that nice, even in the Christian schools. There were girls who I chatted with during the day, but no one who I hung out with outside of the PCS doors. They had their established friends, and their families had their established friendships with the other families. As the new kid, I felt like trying to fit myself into a puzzle that already had all its pieces—a difficult challenge, but this was my first time in any type of environment outside of a church. I didn't know how to insert myself into a high school clique as a newcomer freshman. Shyness and fear of rejection prevented me from putting myself completely into the mix of the other students. Again, I relied on God to bring friends to me. I read my Bible every night and prayed—begging God for a friend. *God has a plan.*

In the winter of my freshman year, the boys in both my class and the upper grades had coined a new term for me—Moses. Yelling at me, "Hi, Moses" every morning. "Hey, Moses! How's it burnin'?" "Hey, Moses? What's up?" I didn't know why they were calling me this, but I didn't care. I was receiving some recognition of my existence, *finally.* I laughed along with them as they used this name for me every day—never hearing them say my real name.

Then the spring of my freshman year, an older girl named Kate, tall and thin with long dirty blonde hair, asked me, "Do you know why they call you Moses?" I looked at her, confused. Her question had caught me off guard because she was popular and had never spoken to me before.

"No. I don't know," I replied.

"You know, Moses and the burning bush?" Kate said in a shushed voice.

Still confused, I looked at her blankly. "Like your *bush*?" she explained. "Because you have red hair! That's all they talk about. How your bush must be red and burning." I stood frozen and shocked! Men had never talked about me or my body in such a demeaning way to my face. How had this happened to me? I dressed modestly every day. I had never flirted or acted in any way that displeased God. I thought I had done everything right, yet a part of my body was being objectified. "Was it my fault?" I wondered frantically. "Did I bring this on myself?" Silently, I kept staring at her, trying to process what she had just said.

"Sorry," she said. "I just felt bad that they kept calling you that, and I kinda realized that you didn't get it." Feeling moronic and realizing the complete sham of the small amount of attention I had received over the last few months, I ran to the bathroom down the hall and cried. Crying and contemplating what to do next, I stayed in the bathroom until I heard Mrs. Hill come in. "Rachel," she said. "Are you in here?"

Mrs. Hill, my Bible class teacher, was a small woman in her mid-forties with short brown hair. She never wore any makeup and always used her class as a platform to discuss the importance of women adhering to traditional biblical values like staying at home to make both dinner and babies. She taught the ninth through eleventh grade Bible classes only, because there might be eighteen-year-olds in the twelfth-grade class, and, as she said, "Once a man is eighteen, a woman has no place teaching him or telling him what he should do. He is a man at eighteen, and godly women are to submit to men and their leadership. 1 Timothy 2:11-14." Mrs. Hill also believed that women should never work outside the home. Of course, she worked outside *her* home by teaching at PCS, but that was deemed okay because it was her ministry.

"Yes. I'm in here," I responded with a tight throat, trying to cover up my tears.

"You're skipping my Bible class," she said in a tone that demanded an explanation.

"CRAP," I thought.

"What are you doing in here?" she continued, as I opened the stall door to meet her steely face with my tear-stained eyes. "You know I'm going to have to give you a detention for this!"

"Mrs. Hill," I began to explain. "I just found out that a group of the boys have been talking about my . . . my um bush and talking about my . . . you know vajayjay and I . . ."

"Rachel," she interrupted. "Boys tease you because they like you. If they didn't touch you, then it's just words. Now come back to class. You're going to have to call your mom on the way to tell her about your detention." I sat in detention that afternoon writing 1 Timothy 2:11-14 over and over again until my one-hour punishment was up: "A woman should learn in quietness and full submission. I do not permit a woman to teach or to assume authority over a man; she must be quiet. For Adam was formed first, then Eve. And Adam was not the one deceived; it was the woman who was deceived and became a sinner."

> Maybe this was my fault? Maybe I had caused
> the boys to sin?

The rest of the year, I remained silent. Every morning I heard, "Hey, Moses! How's it burning?" followed by their giggles. Then I would say a little prayer, "God, give me strength," and continue walking, pretending to be unfazed. "These are just words," I'd remind myself. "The boys are just flirting." I began wearing baggy T-shirts and loose-fitting jeans in an attempt to hide my curvy figure. Trying to push away my other constant, deep-down thought: "If these are just words, why do they feel so violating? Is this my fault?" Before the year had ended, I found one ally. I began to spend most lunch hours with a girl named Riley who had welcomed me to eat with her.

Summer came and went too quickly as it always does in

Portage, where the cold winter months seem never-ending, and the warm summer days are few and far between. Before I knew it, August had come again. Time to go back to school, to PCS. Summer had been meaningful though, as I had met my first-ever boyfriend. All summer I had spent every day with Cory. Cory was Riley's boyfriend's cousin. He had joined them for a soccer game before the end of the previous school year. He noticed me at the soccer game, we hit it off, and before I knew it, I had a boyfriend. He gave me the attention I had been craving since our move to Indiana. Spending every day together all summer became my high. I relied on him to build my confidence and found my worth in him as he reaffirmed my beauty every time we spoke. Even though he didn't go to PCS, I felt less anxious about entering my sophomore year there, knowing I had his love.

As Mom dropped Sarah and me off that August Monday morning to begin our second year at PCS, I felt a little panic, but I was also hopeful that the boys would have moved on to another victim. The first few weeks went fine. I flew under the radar and only heard a boy call me Moses once or twice. The year before, I'd hear them calling me that multiple times a day, so I easily ignored the rare occurrences this year. Every day I went to school, made small talk with a few girls I finally met, including Riley, and worked diligently to be the best in my classes. After school, I headed straight to the YMCA for my job as a lifeguard. This was my life that year. I was content for a while.

In December, I sat in my Bible class, listening intently as Mrs. Hill spoke, when the girl next to me handed me a note. "Who's this from?" I whispered. She just shrugged her shoulders and continued to doodle flowers and hearts on her Bible class worksheet for the day. I put the note in my lap, attempting to hide it from Mrs. Hill while I read it during her class. The front of the note read, "Just wanted you to know . . . " As I opened the note to read the message inside, I began to shake: "You should quit your job as a lifeguard because your legs look like cottage cheese—white and chunky."

I looked up from my lap, trying to control my tears but realized that I couldn't. I quickly stood up and walked out of the classroom without asking permission, my gaze not leaving the floor until I made it to the bathroom down the hall. I ran to a stall and locked myself inside so no one could see me break down in sobs. Until this point, I had always been confident with my body. A negative view of my body had never even crossed my mind. "How could someone send me such a cruel note?" I thought. "What should I do? Is it true? Am I crazy? Did I not dress modestly enough? How I see myself in the mirror must be a lie. The note must be true. Why else would someone write it?" I sat in the stall for the next several minutes, flipping through these questions in my head. The door to the bathroom swung open. It was Mrs. Hill in her navy blue skirt and matching navy blue floral long sleeve blouse. "Rachel, are you in here?"

It felt like bad déjà vu. "Yes," I answered.

"Why did you walk out of my class like that? What do you think you're doing?" Before she could continue, I opened the stall door with bloodshot eyes. This was last year all over again. I cut off her questions by handing her the note. She read it and looked at me. "Who gave you this?" I told her I didn't know.

"I'm sorry that this upset you, but it's just words. Remember, we talked about this last year. Boys will be boys, Rachel! Now clean yourself up and come back to class. You're going to have to stay for detention again today. I can't let you set an example of running out of my classroom like this."

I stared at her, astonished. Why was I going to detention again for something someone else did to me?

When she brought me to the office to call my mom and tell her that I had detention, I saw Principal Rumble. This was my chance. He must understand what had happened and stop Mrs. Hill from giving me detention. I put the phone down and said, "Mr. Rumble, can I please speak with you now?"

Taken aback, Mrs. Hill added, "We would both like to speak with you, Mr. Rumble." Entering his office together, we sat facing him as he sat in authority behind his desk. He had a small office—just big enough for a meeting with two parents. There was framed artwork by children hung up on the walls. I assumed his own children had made these paintings for him. Next to every piece of art, hung a corresponding framed Bible verse. I sat there and began to describe what had happened that day, but I also told him what had happened the previous year with "Moses." I also told him that two boys from the group who had called me "Moses" were in my Bible class and that I was certain one of them had written the note.

He cut me off there. "Rachel. I'm sorry that someone gave you that note, but you can't make assumptions about who gave it to you. You need to be stronger than this. Boys will be boys. They didn't mean anything by it. God tests us in ways that don't always make sense so that we can become stronger in our faith in Him." *God has a plan. God will give you strength.*

"Yes," Mrs. Hill agreed. "That's what I tried to tell her last year and just now." Baffled by the nonchalant attitude of both Mr. Rumble and Mrs. Hill, I sat in his office at a loss for words. Before I could say another word, Mrs. Hill grabbed my hand and said, "Time to go back to class. I'm sure it's a zoo in there because I had to come find you."

"Rachel," Mr. Rumble added as we walked out of his office. "Don't doubt that God will give you strength." I sat in detention that afternoon writing the same verse I wrote the year before, over and over again, until my one-hour punishment ended.

That night I told my parents what had happened earlier in the day and last year, as we ate dinner in our red-and-white kitchen. Mom and Dad both agreed that they were sorry this had happened but "boys will be boys" (how many times can you hear this

43

in a day?) and "boys don't know how to flirt, so they're mean. It's natural." We all prayed together during dinner that I would put my trust in God and that he would give me strength to overcome the words that were thrown at me. *God will give you strength.*

Almost every day for the rest of the year, I received notes in my locker from that group of boys. I knew the group behind the "anonymous" notes because they started addressing all of them with "Moses." They stood in a circle almost every morning waiting for me to open my locker and then giggled as they watched me open my new note. The notes would range from "Have you quit being a lifeguard yet?" to "Why would someone as ugly as you even try to show off your legs?" These messages were more frequent on chapel days, when all of the girls had to wear skirts or dresses to school. I prayed to God every time I received another note that I would be strong and have faith in Him to make me more obedient, but He never stopped my pain. Each day, my confidence felt drained. I actually began to believe what they were saying about me. I kept waiting for God to deliver me from how terrible it made me feel.

During the spring of my sophomore year, I claimed to be sick every day. I couldn't go back into the building to find another note about how disgusting my body looked to other people. After a few weeks being "sick" one or two days a week, Mom finally asked me, "Honey, what is going on?" As I lay in my bed under my neon polka dot comforter, I began to tell her about all the notes that I received and that I had been praying for faith in God, but that I felt "so hurt" and "ugly." My mother sat on my bed and listened intently while I told her what had been going on. After I finished explaining why I didn't want to go to school, Mom said, "Well, Rach, I'm so sorry this has been happening. I had no idea. I thought this was a one-time thing earlier in the year . . . and I don't know what to do. God told Dad and I to send you to this school for a reason, and God hasn't spoken to us yet about moving you to a new school, so we need to pray and ask Him what to do."

That evening, my parents invited two other sets of parents from their Bible study over to pray. They prayed together for hours, asking God where they should send Sarah and me to school the following year, asking Him to reveal his plan to them, asking Him to give them faith. After about two hours of their prayer meeting, Mom and Dad came upstairs to my room where Sarah and I were instructed to sit and do homework while they prayed. They told us that God had spoken to them. *God's truth—the final truth.* He had revealed His plan to them. His plan for Sarah and me was to attend public school in the fall. Mom and Dad added that God had assured them that we would be protected there.

Sarah was "stoked" for the new school. She told Mom and Dad her excitement came the fact that she would *finally* be able to take Mandarin classes, but privately admitted to me that she was excited for an environment with "less rules" and more room for her to showcase her bold fashion choices (like wearing a tie with her button down shirts, which had been frowned upon at PCS for being too "masculine"). As Sarah eagerly shared her excitement with me, I silently thought, "Maybe this was the deliverance I had begged God for?" A wash of relief softened my body. *God's Blessings.*

Courting

I met Cory, my first boyfriend, when I was fourteen. We started dating the summer before my sophomore year at Portage Christian School. When we met, I knew nothing at all about having a boyfriend or a relationship. All I knew was that dating was not allowed in our house and that all relationships required "courting" (courtesy of Joshua Harris and his book, *I Kissed Dating Goodbye*).

At the age of twelve (in order to enforce the standards early on), Mom and Dad explained to me that courting differs from dating in that dating means a lot of one-on-one time together. Courting enthusiasts (including the church and my parents) believe that all romantic relationships should involve group dates with friends and family. Courting is a way to ensure that both parties remain pure until marriage and do not grant themselves the temptation of sexual pleasure (because you are always surrounded by *people*). Also, courting allows your friends and family to get to know the person you are courting and provide their approval or disapproval for marriage—because the end goal of a romantic relationship *is* marriage. In theory, a good Christian woman should marry the first man she courts because leading up to the relationship, both parties have been so diligent in their prayers for God's guidance that neither person enters the courtship without God's blessing for their potential marriage (no pressure). *The blessings of a godly husband.* I mean, what is your worth as a woman if you aren't married by twenty-five?

Cory was my first boyfriend and my first kiss. I was fourteen; he was sixteen. Our "courting" consisted of movie dates with my parents, group dates to the Steak 'n Shake, and spending a lot of time at church. He came from a troubled home where his mom kicked him out of their trailer when he was only fifteen. At that point, he went to live with his estranged father in an attempt to live with some semblance of a family. Unlike some guys, he didn't mind that courting me meant extended time with my family in a stable home environment.

He was not a Christian per se, but since my parents' number one requirement for allowing a guy to date their daughters is Christianity, he claimed to be a Christian and even attended church with my family to strengthen his lie. I think about this piece of my dating history frequently. I constantly imagine how different my younger relationships would have been if Mom and Dad had shifted their energy to the quality of my boyfriends instead of obsessing over their religious name tags. All throughout my dating life, my parents' first question whenever I tell them about anyone I date has been, "But is he a Christian?" They have never asked me, "Does he treat you with respect?" "Does he excite you?" "Do you communicate well?" In their minds, all that matters in a partner is that he's a Christian because Christian men can do no harm. As I think of my parents, I wonder what would have changed in my life if the conversation during my adolescence had been, "This is how you should be treated and treat your partner" in contrast to "DO NOT HAVE SEX BEFORE MARRIAGE" and "only court Christian men." Maybe I would have developed healthy relationship boundaries at a much younger age. Maybe I would have experienced a lot less pain from men too.

Even though courting made it difficult for Cory and me to find alone time together, we were teenagers and always managed to find five or ten minutes alone. We offered to drive to the store when my mom needed something. We would linger in the parking lot to make out before returning home. Sometimes Cory picked me up from school, and we told my parents that we were going to stop for ice cream. His desire and hunger for me provided comfort during all the bullying I endured at PCS. Even though I never directly told him about the bullying (due to shame), he constantly reassured me that I was beautiful—that I was wanted.

Toward the end of our relationship, Cory got antsy for more

than just a hot parking lot make-out session. One day, about two weeks before we broke up, we were sitting in Cory's burnt red rusty '90s station wagon, making out before walking into church. Suddenly, he pulled away. Looking me right in the eyes, he grabbed my hand, and said, "I love you so much. You know that. So um, all the other guys in the youth group say that they feel closer to their girlfriends when their girlfriends, ya know . . . give them blowjobs. Will you give me one, so we can feel closer?"

I sat there in shock, not sure what to say. I didn't know what a blowjob was. I only knew about intercourse and kissing. I also knew that anything outside of the realm of kissing was considered a sin. I looked down at my silver purity ring on my left wedding ring finger, embarrassed, and sheepishly said, "Can you tell me what that is?" He explained what he wanted from me. I thought silently for what seemed like ten minutes. Finally, looking into his eyes, I said, "I don't want to break my promise to purity for my future husband. That sounds like I would be breaking it."

Two weeks later, I broke up with him because a church friend decided to fulfill Cory's previously unfulfilled request for the blowjob in his station wagon. When I found out, I felt betrayed for "honoring God." I thought that purity made me a prized possession for a godly husband. Why did honoring God mean I was now alone?

The Unknown and Unholy Orgasm

After God revealed His will to Mom and Dad for me and Sarah to leave PCS, I entered public school as a junior. Just like before, I entered my junior year knowing no one at Portage High, but, unlike my years at PCS, this time I felt determined to insert myself into social circles. I refused to let my own fear of exclusion get in the way of possible new friendships. In my second week at Portage High, I leaped outside my comfort zone and auditioned for the fall production of *Our Town*.

I heard about the play during my English class one morning. My AP English teacher, Mr. Moody, who quickly fascinated me with his progressive mindset and provocative views on literature, announced before the bell rang, "Don't forget! Fall play auditions are today after school in the auditorium." I immediately perked up—this was my opportunity to not only meet new people but to finally be in a real theater production! When I saw *Footloose* at a local high school while living in St. Simons, I had fallen in love with the theater. The dancing, the music, the story, the characters, the set, the entire production ignited a passion in me that I had never experienced before. Since then, my parents had taken me to many Broadway shows in Chicago including *Wicked*, *The Phantom of the Opera*, and *Joseph and The Amazing Technicolor Dreamcoat*. With each show, I fell more madly in love with the theatre. To this day, the way a show can fill a person so empathetically with joy or sadness captivates me—the theater is where I found myself and will always be my first love.

With enthusiasm, I called Mom after school to tell her I would be late returning home because I had a play audition! She squealed with excitement stating, "Oh, wonderful! I am so glad you are doing this." I think she felt relief in this moment. There was a possibility that her daughter might be able to thrive in her new school—that the experience at PCS would not hold me back.

"Well, I'm really proud of you." She continued, "Sarah needs to go to the audition, too, because I can't come to the school twice this afternoon. She should be fine with that. Just call me when the audition is over, and I'll come grab you gals. Ahh! I can't wait to hear about it!"

Sarah, whose passion for the theater has always matched mine, gladly accompanied me to the auditorium and auditioned herself before I took the stage for my own reading. I stood on the vast empty stage that afternoon, in the audience of Mr. Moody and Mr. Stephens (the theater director), fearlessly reading what every girl had read that afternoon—four lines from the female lead's final heart wrenching speech. Standing there on the stage, I felt more self-assured then I had in years. Instantly, the theatre became home, and the stage became the most familiar place I had ever stood.

The following morning, I ran to the theater door to see if my name appeared on the final cast list for the play. I got there just as Mr. Moody posted the paper. Before I could even search for my name, he looked at me with a smile and said, "Congratulations. You're going to make a fabulous Emily." Then, with a pat on my back, he turned and walked away. Having had no previous acting experience, I was completely shocked when he told me I would be playing Emily, the lead character in this classic play. Although I wanted the lead role, I knew realistically that I had no prior stage experience. After my audition, I thought at best I may be cast for an extra in the graveyard scene. In no way did I ever imagine being cast as the female lead!

At Portage Christian School, we had a "musical" every year, but the musical was always written by students and had to include a storyline of evangelical students saving other students from hell. The choir, including me and my sister, Sarah, would wear matching tie-dye T-shirts and sing a Christian song in between the painfully bad scenes that my fellow students had written. So you can understand my excitement when I found out I would be acting in a REAL play by a REAL playwright. Besides the thrill of being on stage, I was also happy that this experience led me to a large group of new friends outside my traditional church friends from youth group.

The friends I made in the theatre during my time at Portage were not churchgoers. They were liberal and forward-thinking, but filled with compassion and kindness. Until this point, I had never had non-Christian friends. My entire life, I had been warned about the dangers of these friendships, that they would "entice you into sin" and "are a wolf in sheep's clothing." But my time in the theatre proved quite the opposite. My new friends carried more Christian core values—grace, love, justice, empathy, compassion—than many of the "Christians" I had known my entire life. I came to admire and respect these students, silently disowning the prejudices I once held against "non-believers." For the first time in my life, I chose friends outside of the church. The theatre gave me a feeling I had never experienced before: freedom. In the theatre, I felt free to be vocal and have my voice be heard. As Mr. Bodnar (the musical director) frequently said during our rehearsals, "The world will try to silence your voice every day. The theatre is where you learn to be loud and how to stand for something."

As I studied the script for the next few months, I began to adore the character I would be playing. The play follows Emily Webb, my character, from 1901 through 1913 when she was age thirteen through age twenty-six. For Act I and Act II, the audience watches Emily's life from her thirteenth birthday to her marriage, and finally to her untimely death during childbirth. During Act III, Emily watches her family as a ghost (Sarah played an excellent graveyard ghost, filling the void stage alongside other thespians posing as ghosts in a graveyard). As a ghost, she realizes the importance of living in the moment, of loving and living life fully.

After three months of daily and sometimes twice-daily rehearsals, November and opening night arrived. The play ran for six performances over the course of two weekends (Mom and Dad came to show their support at every show), but I remember my opening night performance the best. Although I was shaking with nerves and anxiety before I came onstage for the first scene, after my first line, everything faded. I became Emily for the next two hours. I recited her final monologue as I slowly danced across the stage, embracing her heartbreak as if it were my own: "Oh, earth, you're too wonderful for anybody to realize you. Do any human beings ever realize life while they live it?—every, every minute? I'm ready to go back (to death). I should have listened to you. That's all human beings are! Just blind people." The show ran perfectly that night. Every actor, every light, every scene, all went exactly as planned. I played my part, and I played it to perfection.

After the performance, all the actors, including me, went back to the green room to change before meeting our family or those who had come to support us. As I looked at myself in the mirror and took the white ribbon out of my long red curly hair, my friend Chrissy came over and sat in the empty chair next to me facing the mirror.

"You were wonderful tonight, Rachel! Really, just amazing," Chrissy applauded as she began to rub the bright pink blush off her cheeks.

"Thank you!" I responded. Watching her remove her heavy stage makeup, I said, "You were great too! Everyone was great! I can't believe we actually did it!"

"You know, my friend came tonight. Do you know Braden?" she asked.

I immediately knew who he was. I had seen Chrissy and Braden talk in the hallways at school. I knew that he had English class right after me because we had passed each other on our way to and from the class. I also knew him because he was super-hot—tan skin, rosy cheeks, and dark brown curly hair that hung slightly in his face. I stood up and turned around so Chrissy could help me unzip my costume, a frumpy calico dress with a high neck and a long hem. "Yes. I know who he is. Why?"

"Well, after tonight, he is, like, really interested in you. He asked me for your number," she said, as she helped me out of my costume. "Do you mind if I give it to him?"

"Are you sure? He really wants my number?" I asked.

"Yes! Come on!" Chrissy said, as we both put our costumes on the hanger in the Green Room. "Let me give him your number!"

I agreed, and before the end of the weekend, Braden had called me on my pink razor flip phone. For the next week, we chatted at school every time we saw each other in the hallways. He called me almost every night. But we didn't have very much in common, so we didn't actually talk about much. Basically he was hot, and I was excited that someone as hot as Braden would be interested in someone like me. I enjoyed the attention. The Sunday night after the final performance of *Our Town,* Braden called me to ask me to the Winter Formal the next weekend.

"Um, well, I don't know if my parents will let me go with a boy that they don't know," I told him. "I have to ask them."

"That's lame! I guess if your parents won't let you go with me, then I'll go with someone else."

Hurt that he would consider going with a different girl and desperate to go to the dance with a guy as hot as Braden, I quickly recanted and told him that my parents would "totally agree."

Staring at the *Our Town* poster I had just hung on the back of my bedroom door, I lay down on my polka dot comforter. I knew my parents would never let me go to a dance with a guy that I hadn't courted, meaning someone they hadn't met or spent time with prior to the dance. After a few minutes, I got up the courage to go to my parents' room next door and ask them about the dance. Maybe they would surprise me.

Knock. Knock. Knock. "Come on in," I heard my mom say in her bubbly voice.

"Hey, Mom and Dad. I have a question for you," I said. They were sitting on the love seat at the end of their bed, watching *The Italian Job.*

"Sure, honey," Dad said, as he paused the movie. "What's on your mind?"

I sat down on the floor in front of them. "My friend Braden asked me to go to the Winter Formal with him next Saturday. So, can I go?" I asked with hesitation.

"Rach, you know we can't agree to this," Dad said, looking down at me with his blue eyes. "The dance is a few days away. That isn't enough time for us to get to know him or his intentions."

"But Dad! He's a really nice guy!" I argued. "And it's just a dance!"

"Honey, no. You need to stick to your original plan. Go in the group with your girlfriends from theatre," Dad said firmly. "That will be fun for you."

That ended the conversation. I knew my parents would never have allowed me to go with him, but at least I asked. Standing up silently, I walked back to my room. As I lay in bed that night, I brainstormed what to do next. I could tell Braden that my parents said no, but then he would go with another girl. I could also just lie and tell him that my parents said yes. How would they find out?

The next day at school, I told Braden that my parents said yes, so we made plans for the Winter Formal that weekend. We would meet at Chrissy's house to take pictures with her and her date. Then we would go to the dance. Braden would take me to the dance, and my parents would never find out.

That Saturday night, all went according to plan. Braden met me at Chrissy's house, and we all took pictures before driving five minutes down the road to the dance. I wore a black A-line dress sprinkled with small silver sequins, which hit right above my knees. Braden wore an all-black suit with a black tie. We looked coordinated, like a couple, and I felt so lucky when we walked into the dance together. Braden and I danced all night. We slow danced, dirty danced, and swing danced, having a blast the whole time. I couldn't stop smiling or laughing. Being there with him made me feel special, but more than being there with him, I felt a thrill that I hadn't ever felt before. I kept thinking, "What is the big deal with my parents?" I couldn't understand why they had been so against me going to the dance with Braden. We weren't smoking pot, drinking, or having sex. We were just dancing together! It was innocent, so I didn't feel guilty for the lie that I had told them.

The next morning, I woke up and went downstairs to check my MySpace before getting ready for church. As I turned on our large family desktop Dell, I was immediately welcomed by a screensaver on the computer that read "BUSTED" on top of a picture of Braden and me from the dance the night before. I knew exactly when this picture had been taken. We were on the dance floor toward the end of the dance. His dark curly hair was wet and stuck to his face from dancing for hours. My straightened hair had regained its natural curls from my sweat. In the telltale picture, my butt was backed up on his pelvis, and we were dancing to "Low" by Flo Rida. I knew when this picture had been taken because, at that moment during the dance, I had looked over and saw Lucas, whose mom was my youth leader, Linda. He must have taken the picture and sent it to my parents.

I sat at the computer, staring at my picture of freedom from the night before, trying to put together the details when Mom and Dad walked down the stairs to where I sat on the computer in our bright red kitchen.

"Like the screensaver?" Dad asked me with anger in his eyes.

"I don't really know what to say." Word by word, my tears began to stream down my face. I hated disappointing my parents, and from my dad's face, I knew he was *very* disappointed.

"That's fine. We know that you lied to us and went to the dance with him," Dad kept talking while my thoughts raced. "We also know that he isn't a Christian, and he's been caught smoking pot at school."

How could they have this information? I didn't even know either of these things, mostly because I had never asked during any of our surface-level conversations.

"You're probably trying to figure out how we know all of this. Well, when Lucas sent me the picture, I called your school police officer to ask about this Braden character," Dad said. "I used my Secret Service agent card, and Officer Troy told me all about your date."

Sitting at the computer chair with my head hanging down and my parents standing above me, I cried and just listened to my father's disappointment in me.

"We made an appointment for you to speak with Linda after church today," Mom said with more understanding. "She's going to take you to her house to talk to you." I knew Mom wasn't mad—I could tell by her voice and the way she looked down while standing behind my father during his cross-examination. But she believed honoring God meant sharing a united front with your husband, even when you don't agree with him. With one hand on my slumped shoulder, Mom said, "Now go upstairs to get ready for church and wash up your face."

For the rest of the morning, my fear kept me silent. I had no idea what Linda had in mind to say to me, but I knew she would also express her disappointment. I didn't know if I could handle one more adult telling me how disappointed they were in me, especially when I didn't believe that I did anything wrong. Sure, I could acknowledge that lying to my parents was wrong, but going to a formal and dancing all night? How was that wrong? Nothing happened. I didn't want to date Braden. I wanted to go to one dance with him. I didn't get into any trouble with drugs, alcohol, or sex. Why was everyone so disappointed in me?

After church, my family stood up, and we all walked down the aisle to meet Linda and her family in the front of the church. I walked behind my parents and sister with my head down in shame. We all made pleasantries, ignoring the real reason I was meeting with Linda. Then Mom and Dad handed me off to her for the afternoon. The encounter reminded me of what I witnessed at the end of the week at elementary school when I watched my friends with divorced parents being handed over to the other parent for the weekend. In that situation, everyone engaged in forced small talk and intentionally ignored the intense feelings around the encounter.

Linda, with her olive skin and shoulder-length black hair with wild curls, put her arm around me as we walked out of the church. "I'm so glad we get to hang out all afternoon," she told me, feigning normalcy when everything about this felt strange.

"Okay," I thought, "Maybe this wouldn't be so bad. Maybe she will understand that I didn't do anything against God's will."

Linda's son, Lucas, and her husband, Mike, had gone to lunch together, so Linda and I could have a "private" conversation at their home. It would have been difficult to have an intimate conversation in their small home. I felt relieved, knowing Lucas and Mike wouldn't be there to listen in. I didn't need any more judgment or disappointment.

On the drive over to Linda's house, I sat in the front passenger seat silent, listening to her drone on about her latest diet, which was "sure to help her lose the large thighs and butt" she had gained over the last five years. Arriving at Linda's house after a short drive, we walked up the old cement steps to the front door of their living room. As soon as we walked in, Linda plopped down on the worn green suede couch, motioning for me to sit next to her. The mood instantly shifted. I knew she planned to change the conversation from school and her diet to the dance the night before as soon as I joined her on the couch. Sitting down on the couch next to her, I grabbed the ivory crocheted pillow from the corner of the couch, putting an unconscious barrier between us by placing the pillow on my lap. Linda looked at me silently, her brown eyes piercing my bright blue ones. I knew she wanted me to talk about the dance, but I didn't have anything to tell her. I did not own this conversation.

"Well, Rachel," she said, after a few moments waiting for me to start the conversation. "Let's talk about the dance."

"I don't really know what you want to talk about," I told her, clutching the handmade pillow in my lap.

"How about we start with what Lucas told me he saw?" she said. "He told me that you were dancing provocatively with that boy. Now, I didn't tell your parents about what I want to talk to you about today. I only told them that you went to the dance with him and lied."

"Um . . . yeah," I started, "I went to the dance with him, and I know I shouldn't have lied but . . ."

Linda interrupted. "I'm not as worried about your lie as I am about the way that Lucas said you were dancing. He said you were grinding on that boy all night!"

"But we were just having fun, and I wore a modest dress! Nothing happened between us, . . . you know . . . sexually," I told her shyly, still clutching the pillow in my lap.

"Rachel. Don't lie to me. I know that the way you were dancing with that boy leads to sexual sin." She began retelling the importance of sexual purity, the stories and sermons I had heard since fifth grade. I tuned her out, only hearing a few phrases like, "God is a jealous lover, madly pursuing you," "You led that boy on," and "What kind of Christian example does this set for your new theatre friends?" Everything she said I had heard before, until she stated with conviction, "I know that you probably had an orgasm on that dance floor!"

Wait! What? I thought. *What is an orgasm? And what the heck is she talking about?*

Linda continued. "I know that dancing the way you did on that dance floor, that boy gave you an orgasm. Rachel, orgasms outside of marriage are a sin. You know this, right?"

I knew dressing provocatively was a sin—I hadn't done that. I knew sex and giving into the pleasures of the flesh were sins—I hadn't done that either. I had only danced! What could I be missing here?

"I don't know what you mean, Linda," I said, as I looked at her inquisitively.

"Rachel, don't lie to me. Did your vagina feel warm and tingly? Did you feel sexually aroused? That is an orgasm!"

Confused, I began to cry. I didn't remember feeling these things, but maybe I had had an orgasm? Maybe I had sinned? Maybe I was sexually promiscuous? Maybe I was unworthy? I had disappointed everyone, even God. *God is worthy. I am unworthy. God is everything. I am nothing.*

Linda moved closer to me and put her hand on my back as I cried. "It's okay, Rach," she said softly as she rubbed my back. "God forgives. His perfection covers our imperfection. Would you like to ask God to forgive you for what you did?"

I kept my head bent, attempting to hide my shame and tears. Then I nodded. Of course I wanted God to forgive me! I didn't want this orgasm to keep me from His perfect will for my life. *The blessings of eternal life. The blessings of joy.* Then we prayed together. Linda asked that God would "protect me from sexual desires" and that he would "guard" my heart. I cried in shame as I asked God to forgive me for my "sexual desires" and my "orgasm." That afternoon I left Linda's house convinced that I had had an orgasm and even more convinced of the sinfulness of female pleasure.

My parents grounded me for the next three months, only allowing me to go to school, the theatre, and church. I never spoke to Braden again, and he never tried to speak to me. I found out a few weeks later that when my dad had called the school police officer, he asked Officer Troy to "scare Braden" from ever speaking to me again. I'm not sure what Officer Troy said to Braden, but whatever he said, it worked.

Kneeling for Christ

Almost as soon as my three-month grounding ended, I met John, a tall, handsome, popular guy, with dark-rimmed glasses, who loved wearing tight clothing that revealed his muscles. John and I shared AP History together all year, but we had never really spoken until one warm spring afternoon. My after-school *Grease* rehearsal had been cancelled, so I left school on time that day, a rarity during theatre rehearsal season. After the final bell sounded, I hastily made my way out to the parking lot, but I didn't make it to my car because a surprising someone stopped me—John. He pulled up next to me, outside the entry doors to our high school in his bright apple red Mustang convertible and said, "Who wants a ride?" I looked around, and there was no one next to me. He was talking to me! Taken aback by his forwardness, I was momentarily at a loss for words. Then I said, "I can take a quick ride."

We drove all around our small-town cornfields with the convertible top down, engaging in conversation. We flirted the whole hour. By the end of the ride, I was attracted to way more than just his obvious good looks. Before we became a couple, he pursued me with dedication for about two weeks bringing me flowers, writing me romantic notes, and walking me to all my classes. What I initially thought was just a flirty fast ride quickly turned into an accelerated relationship.

When John asked me if I would be his girlfriend, I immediately said yes. Then I explained to him that my response actually depended on my family's response and that John needed my father's permission to date me before I could be his girlfriend. John thought this was strange but agreed to the rule because, as he said, "I would do anything for you." That night John came over to my house and was immediately greeted by my dad (who reached the front door before me). Dad, a six foot tall Secret Service agent with a head shaved as smooth as Mr. Clean's, welcomed John to join him alone in the kitchen.

They both sat at the kitchen table together as Dad explained our severe family courting rules and the expectation that John would come to church every Sunday. Dad delivered this speech with a rifle in his hand, so he could assert his power as my father and his ownership over me. "Now, John," he said standing eye to eye with him in our kitchen, "I want you to know that Rachel is a gift from God. She has made a purity promise to both me and the Lord that she will wait until marriage for any type of sexual funny business, so don't make me use this rifle on you." Then he laughed and invited John to play basketball with him in our front driveway. I waited inside, mortified that Dad acted this protectively and terrified that John would speed away from me at any moment.

Peeking out the front window a few times, I saw them laughing together as John deliberately took it easy on my dad, who, despite his knee problems, thought he was twenty-three. I still have no idea what they talked about as they played basketball, but when they returned, John stunned me. He wanted to court me, even after this incredibly awkward conversation with my father.

Although I could not see most of John's reactions that night, he later told me with a laugh that he "made it out alive" and that he would wear my dad's approval as a "badge of honor." He went above and beyond to call me his girlfriend. It felt like my own fairy tale.

At the start of our relationship, we spent a lot of time at John's house doing "homework." He lived with his single mom, who worked full time at Sears Hardware. After school, we always had the house to ourselves. My parents were completely unaware that we had this time alone. With this secret freedom, our physical relationship took off quickly. We were sixteen with raging hormones.

One evening, a week or so before summer break began, John began driving me back to my house after we had hung out with our friends at Steak 'n Shake all night. I looked at the clock in his car— 9:00 p.m. I needed to be home by 10:00 p.m. "I have plenty of time," I thought with relief. On our drive to my house, John made an unexpected turn into the desolate library parking lot. He put the car in park and looked at me as he said, "Since you don't have to be home for a little while longer, let's spend the rest of our night alone." Then he unclipped his seat belt and leaned over so our lips gently touched. We began kissing passionately and, shortly into our detour, his right hand started unbuttoning my khaki Hollister shorts. Defensively, I pulled his hand away, looked down and said, "I can't have sex until marriage . . . I um . . . I'm sorry." *My value is virginity. Sex outside of marriage will leave me alone.* He put his hand under my chin and pulled my face up to look into his eyes. Giggling, he said, "I'm not having sex with you. I'm making you feel good."

Growing up in the Evangelical Christian world, my church and my parents limited my knowledge of sex and pleasure. They taught me to live my life by these certain "facts": "Sex is only for marriage between a man and a woman . . . Sex before marriage will leave you in pieces, and no man wants a woman who isn't whole for him . . . Sex will only feel pleasurable in the context of marriage . . . Women don't think about sex unless they want to please their husband." I honestly knew nothing else about sexuality besides these "truths" the church and my family gave me. No one ever discussed the instinctual nature of sex, the consensual nature of sex, or the beauty of the act itself. At that time, I thought the sole purpose was to pleasure a man, specifically a husband, and to bear the "fruit" (aka children). I had also been told, over and over again, about the sinfulness of the act outside the context of marriage.

When I started dating John, I had very limited knowledge about foreplay. I had only heard Corey's explanation about blow-jobs. I didn't know that women could feel pleasure from sex or that foreplay for women even existed. My entire knowledge of sex had revolved around what sex meant for men. The idea of embracing and celebrating women's bodies and our sexuality had never been recognized or discussed. I believed what the church had taught me— sex is meant to be pleasurable for men. Women will receive pleasure when they see their partner pleasured.

That night, I realized the errors in my sexual knowledge. I learned how good it felt to be pleasured. As John moved my khaki shorts and Victoria Secret cotton underwear down my legs to the floor of the car, my entire body began to tingle. My body was silently screaming for his touch. He slowly began to caress my clit as he moved one finger, then another, into my vagina. His fingers went in and out of me quickly as his thumb continued to circle my clit. I had never felt anything like this. Captivated in that moment, I closed my eyes as my breath began to quicken. My body began to rhythmically contract and shake until *ahhhh*. Happy sigh. "WHAT WAS THAT?" I thought, as I noticed the smell of damp summer grass drifting through the car windows. I had never felt anything like that, my being solely focused on sensation and pleasure. My body felt a euphoria it had never experienced before, and, honestly, in that moment, sin was the farthest thing from my mind. I wanted that feeling, that experience to happen again and again.

After I finished, I began to pull my shorts up from my ankles, expecting John to start the car and take me home. Instead, he looked at me and asked, "Now will you do that for me?"

Hesitant, I replied, "Um . . . I've never done this before."

"I'll tell you what I like," he said with assurance. He unzipped his cargo shorts as I zipped my shorts back on. Grabbing my hand, he placed it on his penis. "Bleeding Heart Baby" by Head Automatica was playing loudly through the cherry red Mustang speakers as he moved my hand up and down his shaft at the speed and tightness that he liked for about thirty seconds. My new-found euphoria disappeared instantly. I felt scared. Was I sinning? I had to be. This was basically sex, right? "Now put your mouth on it and suck," he said. I did what he told me but couldn't let him enter my mouth very deeply without gagging and losing my ability to breathe. Luckily, he came in my mouth within a few seconds, releasing me from this duty as soon as I swallowed his cum. Swallowing seemed like the quickest way to get rid of the shame his taste made me feel. Honestly, I didn't know what else to do with it. He zipped up his pants and leaned over to kiss the top of my head before starting the car and heading back to my house.

When I walked inside, my parents asked how my night was. "Good," I said, "but I'm tired." I went straight to my room up the stairs, hoping that they wouldn't ask me any other questions. I lay on my bed and cried. I wasn't sure what had happened that night, but I knew it felt too good to be something that could be holy. *My value is virginity. Sex outside of marriage will leave me alone.* My head began to swarm with questions and doubts. Was that the orgasm Linda warned me about? Was I impure now? Would I have to shamefully tell my future husband about this? Would any man want me now that I had given a piece of myself to John? I wasn't sure, but I was certain I couldn't talk to anyone about it.

We entered our senior year of high school very much in love and in a deep exploration of each other's bodies, despite only dating for about six months. During this time, John had become involved with my family's church but still did not claim to be a Christian. Our youth pastor, Linda, continuously worked overtime to convert John to Christianity, according to my parents' request. She even had a church donor pay for his youth retreat registration so that he had no excuse to not attend. We went together. By the end of the retreat, he confessed his sins to God and became a born-again Christian. My parents and Linda were thrilled. So was I. His Christianity meant our relationship now honored both my parents and God, so these were two sins I no longer had to confess nightly. We saved his soul, which meant my parents would finally fully accept him. His salvation seemed like a win for everyone.

Shortly after this retreat, John confronted me. He told me that he had prayed to God and spoken to Linda about our sexual relationship. I sat in alarmed shock. I never told anyone what happened between us because I knew they would judge us. For him to tell the youth pastor so quickly after his conversion startled me. He said we should stop all physical touch besides kissing because any type of intimacy outside of kissing is "unholy" and "sinful." Linda had also promised him that if we "stopped," she wouldn't tell my parents because "God would forgive us."

"Linda explained that you should never have let our relationship become so physical," he told me. "You are the Christian! In order for us to move forward in God's will, you will have to repent for drawing me into sin before I became a Christian." He was right. The sexual encounters were my fault. I shouldn't have caused him to fall into sinful patterns. I shouldn't have seduced him. My desires and my body caused this. *My value is virginity. Sex outside of marriage will leave me abandoned.*

Our abstinence lasted about two months before we were naked in bed together again—never having intercourse though . . . this was our hard stop. That afternoon, we began making out, which led to him asking for a blowjob. I obliged and then asked for him to go down on me. "I really don't think that honors God," he said. "In fact, you should never have given me a blowjob. You should have been stronger for both of us. I'm still learning this Christian stuff." With tears in my eyes, I quickly got dressed and kneeled next to his cum-stained, navy blue comforter. I prayed for forgiveness from God while John began the mundane task of his homework. The encounter was entirely my fault; I had sinned for both of us.

Two weeks later we were at his mom's house again, doing our homework, when he said, "I'm really worried . . . I just don't feel like you love me. I need you to make me feel like you love me." Desperate to keep him and feel worthy of his love, I kneeled and unzipped his pants. He touched no part of my body and made no effort to. I played the part of the vessel in a transactional experience for his pleasure. As soon as he finished, he again told me that we had sinned and that the encounter was my fault.

During our senior year of high school, John applied to Indiana University. Although I knew nothing about Indiana University, I followed suit in order to be close to him. We both received early acceptance due to our high school GPAs, so we were able to spend the majority of our last year in high school daydreaming together about what our future at IU would hold. I would study premed; John would study business. We both had high career aspirations and felt as though we could conquer anything if only we had each other. John and I were both so excited for our new college adventure together that before we headed off to college, we even got matching cross tattoos (mine on my left foot and his on his back), to symbolize our commitment to God and our love for each other.

It was August 2009. My parents' car was packed to the brim with all my college essentials. Mom and Dad had agreed to send me to a public university under two stipulations: I must immediately become involved in the Campus Crusade for Christ ministry on campus, and I must become a member of a church within the first two months. This was their rationale to my dad's sister, who told him that I was "stepping into sin" and "opening my heart to the devil" by attending a public university over a Christian university, which all her children had attended.

Mom and Dad moved me into my new dorm room. We all shed a few tears before they headed back north to Portage. During our goodbyes, Mom said, "Honey, we are so proud of you!" Then Dad chimed in: "You are going to do great things here!" I cried as we exchanged hugs and felt their hope for my next journey. Unfortunately, I did not hold onto that hope for long. Within one day outside of my parents' strict supervision, John had again manipulated me into making him "feel good," then forced me to repent to God. I remember this afternoon specifically because it had been almost a year of this pattern. I was exhausted. Looking at him, I asked with desperation, "Will you please touch me?"

"No, your . . . *that* . . ." he said, motioning to my vagina, "is dirty. Why are you trying to make me sin?" I felt his hatred for my body deeply. I began to hate myself as well and did what I could to control my life. At the time, that meant regulating and deeply limiting my food intake. I was frail on the outside and wounded on the inside. John made a job of manipulating our religion and my desire to please him to his personal sexual satisfaction. He had given me a taste of what my body could enjoy and the pleasure it could feel. Then he took it away from me completely in the name of God. Since John became a Christian, when he asked for his pleasure, I always told him "No," but my voice never seemed loud enough. "No" went nowhere with John. He knew how to make me concede. "You don't love me," he would say. Or "If you don't love me, then I will leave you." With those words, he coerced me into "Yes" every time.

This cycle of abuse and manipulation worsened over the course of our freshman year at Indiana University. John and I both became very involved in Campus Crusade for Christ, as I agreed to do with Mom and Dad. Our gender-specific bible studies led to more shame and guilt but did not lessen instinctual sexual desire. Every week, I met with this group of women in the lobby of the Teter dorm. We discussed our time since we last met, how we could pray for one another, and read a small passage of scripture. I never asked for prayer for anything regarding my relationship. No one could know what was happening with John because it was my body and my sin that caused it. John, however, frequently told his all-male Bible study that I had caused him to "sin" and that I constantly tried to seduce him. He told me that the men in his Bible study prayed together for God to give John the "strength to say no" and that God would eliminate my sexual desires until marriage. He liked to remind me of this as he watched me pray after he demanded his sexual gratification from me.

I never spoke to anyone in my Bible study or anyone from our church about what was happening because sex and sexuality were taboo. I knew that if I shared our encounters with anyone, I would again be told that this was my fault for causing John to sin. It was my fault because, as a woman, it was my job to not allow men to desire me sexually. At that time, I truly believed that what was happening was my fault. My body was a vessel of sexuality that caused men to sin. It was something that required my repentance. This "truth" goes as far back as the small red book and Mom buying me my first bra.

Everything else with John seemed wonderful in my mind. He loved God. Check. He loved me. Check. My parents loved him. Check. I loved his parents. Check. We had the same friend group. Check. He pushed me to be a better Christian by requiring me to go to church and Campus Crusade with him every week. Check.

By January of our freshman year, I made up my mind—John needed to propose, and we needed to get married. This was the only option. It would eliminate all guilt, shame, and abuse because sexuality within marriage is God's plan. *God's Blessings.* We couldn't break up because what other Christian man would want to unwrap a damaged present? John was good at being nice in public—as most abusers are. I thought that no one would ever even believe me if I told them what happened behind closed doors. I felt trapped. I thought God would take all this shame and guilt away if we entered into His holy covenant. Our relationship would finally be perfect because I had checked every box except the one for sex. Before we returned to school for our second semester, I told John that I believed it was in God's plan for us to get married. John agreed, and on my nineteenth birthday, he proposed.

The proposal was what women dream of and what you read about in wedding magazines. It was a warm and sunny day on the

Lake Michigan beach near our homes. John brought his guitar and sang a song he wrote for me to the tune of Jack Johnson's "Better Together." He had rewritten the lyrics to match our love story. After the song, he bent down on one knee and asked me to marry him with my Nana's engagement ring. I cried happy tears of relief. The shame and guilt would soon be over. I was going to be married; everything was going to be better. I would no longer be a sinful woman in the eyes of God. John may have taken off some of the wrapping my beautiful present of virginity, but he would be the only man I would ever be with, so God had to forgive me. Being married meant that God would finally approve of my sexuality.

We spent the rest of our summer planning our wedding and attending pre-marriage counseling at our church. We had one pre-marriage counseling session together in a small church office with navy blue walls and a framed certificate of Pastor Tim's ministry degree from Moody Bible Institute in Chicago. After making pleasantries, Tim immediately asked, "Do you believe in birth control?"

"Yes," I said firmly. "I'm nineteen and need to finish college. Also, being a mother is the furthest thing from my mind right now." I stared into the only picture on his desk, which featured himself, his wife, and their four children (all very close in age).

The pastor looked at John and asked, "What do you think about this?"

"I want to follow Christ in marriage, so I will do what he tells us," John said.

Our pastor sighed and was silent for a moment before looking straight into my eyes. "Sex is not for your pleasure, Rachel," he said severely. "It is for John and for you all to start a family. Birth control should not be something you are considering because it is not in God's natural plan. How could it be? There is no faith there."

I sat silently as the pastor spoke for the rest of our session about the evils of birth control and sexual desire. Ironically, John said that he agreed with the pastor and wanted to be a God-honoring husband. A "God-honoring husband" that sexually abuses and manipulates his fiancée?

At the end of our session, our pastor asked that John come alone for the next session. The following week, John met with Pastor Tim. Then he came over to my parents' house afterward. John and I sat on my parents' front porch so we could have a somewhat private conversation. He told me that Pastor Tim had shared his concerns with John about who I was as a person. Pastor Tim had told him that he believed I was too "independent" and "self-minded" to be able to enter a godly marriage where the woman should "submit to her husband daily." John told me that I needed to begin submitting to him if I wanted him to marry me. He said I needed to "honor him like I would honor and serve Christ." I agreed. I couldn't argue with John or our pastor. I was the problem. I must have been.

Going back to Bloomington that fall for our sophomore year, I was thrilled because, after a difficult application process, I had been chosen to be a resident assistant at Wright Dorm. John would be living about ten minutes off campus with a group of five guys from his Bible study. I would be living on campus while I worked as an RA. I hoped that since we were not living a five-minute walk from one another, like the year before, and since he would be living with five Christian dudes, that we would be able to abstain from any sexual sin for the entire school year until our wedding the following summer. However, we were unable to abstain that year.

Living in a dorm room by myself meant that John came over almost every night, but he would never spend the night because then his Christian roommates would assume that we were stumbling into sin. He would come over, ignore my "No" and coerce me for his pleasure. Then he would leave, kissing me on the forehead before exiting and saying, "I love you so much." I slept alone every night, forced to wrestle with all of the hate that I felt toward myself. With all this stress, I ate even less than the year before. I was a transparent ghost: no voice, no independence, and no freedom. I felt filled with so much contempt for who I was. To continue going before God to ask for forgiveness and make promises I could not keep crippled me.

In place of their first meeting of the year, Campus Crusade

threw a big welcome back to campus party. The meeting was held on campus in Woodburn Hall, where I had my anatomy lecture on Tuesday and Thursday mornings the year before. Woodburn Hall seats almost 200 students. Since it had been advertised on flyers to all the non-Christian students as a "campus party," that first meeting was jam packed.

We started with the normal opening games and icebreakers to get everyone laughing and talking. Then we were called back to take our seats by John's roommate, Remy, who was leading the meeting that evening. He welcomed us back to campus and added, "A dear friend who is also one of my roommates is going to come up here and tell us about how influential Campus Crusade has been in his life over that last three years at IU. Let's give it up for Trevor."

Trevor walked up to the lecture stage where Professor Lundin taught me anatomy (a class I had loved) twice a week for the entire semester before. Trevor was tall and gangly, with large thick-rimmed glasses that swallowed his face. He had on a muted plaid button-down shirt and khaki pants. Remy handed the microphone to him. I sat silently next to John as he began to give his testimony, disguised as his experience with Campus Crusade, so that the non-Christians there would stay and listen.

I had known Trevor my entire time at IU. He was in John's Bible study the year before and was now one of his roommates. His girlfriend was also an RA on staff with me at Wright. Looking at Trevor, it was nice to see a familiar face in a room of 200 people. Trevor's temples dripped large clear beads of sweat as he took the microphone from Remy. I could clearly see his pit stains from my seat in the back of the lecture hall. Trevor started with pleasantries about the community he had found through Campus Crusade and the lifelong friends he had made, but the evening quickly took a dark turn when he said, "Everyone here has been with me, even as I have struggled with my sexuality." What was he saying? I didn't understand. He continued. "Last year, my girlfriend, Staci, read my journal that I keep under my bed. In it, she found . . ." Trevor stopped and took a deep breath as his eyes watered up. "She found my fantasies written onto paper. My fantasies with men."

Shocked, I remember asking myself, "What happens now?" I had never known a gay person, let alone a gay "Christian." Trevor went on to explain that he had kissed a man before and had always been attracted to men, but that it was God's will for him to live his life in a mixed-orientation relationship and soon marriage. Staci had forgiven him. They prayed nightly together for Trevor to resist his urges. He ended with "God is good. The life He has planned for me is great. I choose to walk in His promise." *The blessings of eternal life.*

I sat silently, unable to move and filled with confusion, as John and all those around me began to stand up, cheering and clapping for Trevor's bravery. Slowly I stood and clapped too because I didn't really know what else to do. I remember this night with sickness in my stomach.

John walked me home that night. "Wow, babe!" he said. "Isn't it amazing what God is doing in Trevor's life?"

Quietly, I responded, "I don't know." This evening was the first time I had to directly think about homosexuality and Christianity. The LGBTQ community was never something my parents talked about in detail. It was never discussed in the churches we attended. When I was younger, I remember one service where the pastor read Romans 1:26-28 and briefly spoke about the evils of "same sex lust," but otherwise, same-sex attraction was a taboo subject, never really mentioned outside of that. I couldn't understand why men loving men or women loving women was considered a sin. No one ever gave me a clear reason why it was considered "sinful." The church simply said, "Well, it isn't *natural.*" In high school, when I had asked my parents about God and homosexuality, they looked quite uncomfortable and explained that marriage is only between a man and a woman, which further confused me. How could love differentiate between sexuality?

John stopped in his place, right in front of the IU Auditorium, and angrily told me, "SEE! This is what Pastor Tim was talking about! You're challenging my authority and the authority of God. How can I marry someone who cannot submit to God's commandments?"

As a tear ran down my face, I looked at the ground, remembering Pastor Tim's words after his private session with John. I was completely run-down. The night had taken all my energy. I had no idea what to think or feel. Scared that John would leave me and that no other man would want anyone as broken as me, I quickly apologized and added, "You're right." Continuing our walk back to my dorm silently, John continued telling me how impressed he was with Trevor's testimony and courage.

That semester, John's verbal abuse became too much for me to bear. It was as though what Pastor Tim had said to John had given him the green light to put me down as often as he deemed necessary in the name of God. Anything he found imperfect about me could be used against me to beat me down even more than he already had sexually. I remember riding in John's bright red Mustang one afternoon after our classes. I was singing Lady Gaga's new song, "Poker Face." Idina Menzel had just covered this song on that week's episode of *Glee*. As a theatre nerd, I became obsessed with Menzel's rendition. I had been singing the song all week, but this was the first John had heard me gleefully belting the song. Right after the first chorus played on his old 64G iPod in his car, John ripped the iPod from the cord that connected it to his speakers. "What is this?" he asked me, speeding up the car.

"It's the new *Glee* cover of 'Poker Face.' Isn't it amazing? I can't stop singing it! You know I saw Idina Menzel in Chicago . . ."

"Why would you ever sing something like that?" he demanded. "It's about weird sex stuff. Lady Gaga isn't anyone who Christian women should be following. She's like gay or something, and her songs are all about drugs and sex."

I had had enough. Even though we were on our way off campus to grab dinner, I asked John to turn around and take me home. His clenched body and pink face revealed his anger. "Why would you want to go home?" he asked me. "We have a date planned." We had never had a fight where I had not immediately apologized to him and prayed. This time would be different. My voice started quietly but began to grow with confidence as I spoke. "I want to go home because you're being mean." My voice climbed louder, "I was having fun, and singing this song makes me happy! You can't tell me what to sing!"

Teeth gritted, he said, "I can't, but God can!"

After John turned the car around, we didn't speak for the entire seven-minute ride back to my dorm. I got out of his car. Neither of us said "Goodbye" or "I love you." I simply walked inside and went straight to my small dorm room.

I had never before challenged John or what he told me. In fact, I had never challenged any man. My parents had always made it very clear that the woman's place is next to men but that men have the final authority on everything. I had seen my dad scream at my mom my whole life. She would always apologize immediately, then pray. I thought this behavior was normal and even healthy. A wife submits to her husband as women are to submit to the Lord. On multiple occasions, Mom said to Sarah and me regarding parental decisions, "I know this isn't fair, but your dad has the final say in any decision when we disagree. It is the way God intended it." Standing up to men was something I didn't know I had the power to do, but with this one moment in John's Mustang, I felt a flash of power stirring inside of me. It felt exhilarating.

In my dorm that night, I went to visit with my fellow RA friends, Sam, a preppy joyful spirit with blond hair, and Hilary, a small-town girl with a wicked sense of humor. That night, we participated in our weekly ritual—watching the new episode of *Glee* together. We were all crammed in tight on Sam's floor in his red-and-black dorm room. My phone would not stop ringing. At this point, John had called me about eleven times. Sam noticed I was ignoring my phone.

"Do you want to get that, Rach?" he asked. "The show doesn't start for five minutes. You have time!"

I didn't want to look out of sorts, so I stepped into the hallway to return John's calls. "Hi. I saw you called . . . What? . . . You're outside? You left two hours ago? . . . Well, we are watching *Glee,* so I don't think you want to come in . . . Okay. I'll come let you in the building." John had returned. He wanted to talk to me about the incident in the car. I told him it would need to wait until after *Glee.* I peeked my head back into Sam's room and asked, "Is it okay if John comes to watch?"

"Sure, but hurry!" Sam replied. "It's starting,"

As John and I took a seat on the floor, Sam and Hilary said hi and John nodded at them in return. Within fifteen minutes, John abruptly got up. "I can't watch this," he said. "I'm leaving." I followed John as I apologetically mouthed the words "I'm SORRY" to Sam and Hilary. In the hallway, John sternly explained that he wanted to talk to me. "I cannot sit there and watch that gay sinful show," he said. Then he stormed out of the building. "I'll call you when I am ready."

Confused and feeling like the power stirring inside me had completely disappeared from my spirit, I walked back into Sam's room. We all finished the episode in silence. I felt mortified by John's outburst, just wanting to pretend like nothing had happened. To everyone around us, we always seemed like the perfect Christian couple. John had just shone a light into the dark backstage view of our relationship.

When the episode ended, Hilary looked at me. "Is everything okay?"

Not missing a beat and with a forced smile, I replied, "Yes. Why?"

Sam hopped on his bed. "John just isn't fun, and you need fun! He's like a potato!"

"I'm just worried about how angry he was," Hilary said. "He just stomped out of here like a toddler."

"I pissed him off today," I said, defending him as I always did. "I'm sorry that he wasn't being social. It's my fault. I'm the one who made him mad." Embarrassed and not ready to discuss the topic any further, I excused myself to my dorm room one hallway away. As soon as I locked myself in my room, my body collapsed on my twin bed. I began to sob, not sure why I felt this amount of exhaustion and distress. I knew, though, that something in my spirit had been wrong for a long time, and I felt it finally breaking. Alone, I curled up into a ball and cried until I fell asleep.

The next morning, I still felt unsettled, but I wasn't sure why. John's anger and his verbal abuse were common occurrences. These had been staples in our relationship since his conversion to Christianity. Why was I now so upset? What made me realize I couldn't survive in this relationship much longer?

I texted him. "Hi. Can you come over after your classes today?" He texted back that he would come over around 4:00 p.m. It was 7:30 a.m., and I had a lecture at 8:00 a.m. I started getting ready for class. As I put on my makeup in my small Ikea dorm room mirror, I dropped my mascara and collapsed on the floor. I wasn't sure what was happening, but I couldn't breathe or move. I was hyperventilating and frozen, my body in a tight ball on the floor. This was my first anxiety attack. I thought I was dying. I lay there, trying to sort out my thoughts, but I couldn't think. What was happening? What had been happening to me for years? Who is this man? Can I marry him? Is God mad at me? Is this all my fault? Am I a failure? Am I happy? NO! And with that last question, finally, my mind could slow down and answer. *Deep breath.*

Okay, let me try another question. When was the last time I felt happy? I couldn't remember. As I admitted this to myself, I clutched my stomach. I could feel all my ribs. I was not well. This was the first time I had felt just how shattered I had become. Shaking and still unable to move off the floor, I came to realize what I needed to do when John came over that afternoon. Skipping all my classes that day, I lay on the floor until I could move to my bed. Then I stayed in my bed until John knocked on my door. Small steps.

Knock. Knock. Knock. My stomach churned. My gut felt as if all its components were begging to be cut out of me. He was here. I rose from my bed and with red swollen eyes, I opened the door. John walked in and casually asked, "Why do you look like that?"

This was the moment. I knew what I had to do. I felt like I had no strength or energy left in my body but remembered the small stirring of power I had experienced a few days before. I knew that I needed every ounce of power I had. I also knew it had been hiding somewhere inside for a long time. I asked him to sit on the twin bed, my hot pink jersey pillow had turned dark red, still soaked from my tears. Standing in front of him, I felt afraid of what might happen when I told him what I had decided.

Earlier that semester, my sociology professor had spoken about Margaret Atwood and the feminist movement, most of which I had ignored. But in this moment, I clearly remembered a quote from Atwood that my professor had written on the board for the class to discuss: "Men are afraid that women will laugh at them. Women are afraid that men will kill them."

In that moment, staring into John's eyes as I stood above him looking down, I remembered these words that I had previously ignored. Nothing rang more true in this moment than the fear coursing through every fiber of my being.

I started with a shaky voice but no tears. "John, we need to talk . . . I am not happy . . . "

"Happiness comes from God," he interrupted, "so you need to pray to Him about this."

"No," I responded, still with no tears. "I'm not happy because of you."

He sat silent. I watched his every movement. He clasped his hands together so tightly they became white. I needed to do this quickly before the courage I had mustered vanished. "We need to call off the wedding. I can't do this with you anymore. I'm so . . . so not okay." There, I had said it.

I was afraid John had cut off the circulation in his hands; he kept them clasped so tight. When he raised his head to look at me, his eyes were full of fire. I took a step back. "Do you really think you can leave ME?" he said. "Who do you think would actually want you? I've put up with you for three years. Do you really think someone else would do that for you?" When he came towards me, he grabbed my arms and pulled my stiff body into his chest. "How can you leave this? How can you leave our love?"

I stood silent and still as a corpse, clasped in a suffocating embrace that prevented me from showing any affection toward John. "I don't know," I finally muttered. "But I'm not happy." Now my tears started flowing again. My eyes seemed like a flooded basement that day. "I don't know why, but I'm not happy. I can't do this anymore."

"Fine!" he snarled, moving to the door. "If this is really what you want, then I'm gonna walk out this door, but I hope that you freaking know that you'll never find anyone who loves you like I do—or treats you as good as I do. I'm the best you'll ever have. You don't even deserve me!"

Looking him in the eyes, I felt the power stirring stronger, allowing me to stand tall. He waited for me to apologize and change my mind as I had done so many times before and for so many years. But as each second went by, my power grew. I stood taller, more sure in my decision. "Fine," he said again as he walked out the door. "Remember what I said. You will never have anything better than me. Ever. Who is going to want YOU?" Then he slammed the door for the last time.

College

"Making women the sexual gatekeepers and telling men they just can't help themselves not only drives home the point that women's sexuality is unnatural, but also sets up a disturbing dynamic in which women are expected to be responsible for men's sexual behavior."

—Jessica Valenti, *The Purity Myth*

You Can't Sit with Us

Ending my engagement with John was the hardest thing I have ever done. To this day, I have no idea where that strength came from or how I had the power to choose myself over a relationship I believed had been appointed by God. I will never forget calling my parents that night and explaining that I had broken up with John, but I gave them no real reason why. When you're in the depth of an abusive and manipulative relationship, I think it's almost impossible for you to use words to explain what happened. Like other abused girls and women, I minimized the breakup for myself and for them, so I didn't have to feel the extent of the trauma I'd been through. "He's just not right for me." "He has a temper." "We fell out of love." "I just wasn't happy." It was easier for me to say, "I realized that we weren't right for each other" because this avoided people's questions or judgments.

That night, although they were confused, Mom and Dad still showed me support. However, I don't think that they really knew how to act or how we would all move forward. They said that they "trusted my choice" and that if "God has appointed John as your husband, you will find your way back to each other at that time. The timing is probably just off." Then they took over canceling our wedding venue and hiding my wedding dress in their closet so I wouldn't have to see it. They also told all our family, including Nana, my Norwegian grandmother who sewed my navy silk shawl for my first Cotillion ball. Even though Mom and Dad did not know the words to comfort me during this time, they showed their love and support by taking on the most difficult part of cancelling a wedding—informing everyone involved and really shielding me from the shame that can come up in those conversations.

A few days later, Nana called me to ask how I was doing. She had this incredible gift of knowing the pain people were experiencing, even if they never verbalized it—almost like she knew how to help people before they could help themselves. I could tell that she didn't believe any of my rehearsed lines about my breakup with John, but she never pried. "God has great plans for you," she told me. Then she asked me to keep her engagement ring, which John had used to propose. Jokingly, she said, "I'm going to die in a few years anyway. What good will that ring do for me? You keep it and remember me by it." The call was short, but before I got off the phone, Nana said that she would love for me to write her weekly letters, telling her about my life. I agreed and sent the first letter that week. Looking back, I see that those letters weren't for her; they were for me. She knew that I could not verbalize the hurt or heartbreak I felt, but I think she hoped that by writing to her, I would begin to heal.

John was out of my life, but that didn't change my desire to honor God and stay involved in Campus Crusade. I knew I needed support from my church community during this time, but I also realized that attending the weekly Campus Crusade meetings might be too difficult for me. I would have to see John every week, something I was not ready to do. Still, I decided that attending my women's-only Bible study would be a safe space. So, the week after we broke up, I went to my Bible study prepared to give my rehearsed response as to why John and I had broken up. I didn't have a lot to say because I really didn't completely understand my decision. I couldn't see the abuse for what it was and had been for many years. I just knew that I had been unhappy for a long time, so this became my excuse.

As we all gathered in the living room making small talk at

Lauren's house, I began to respond to all the girls' questions with my prepared response: "I just wasn't happy and hadn't been in a long time." Everyone respected my answer, except my two Bible study leaders, Lauren and Tatum. Lauren, an incredibly thin woman with long dark brown hair and large brown eyes, came up to me after our meeting. While everyone began to leave, she asked, "Are you doing okay?"

"I'm just really sad and lonely. I hope I made the right decision because my heart hurts," I replied, feeling vulnerable.

Tatum came over to Lauren's blue couch and moved a white decorative Colts pillow so she could sit on the other side of me. She was also extremely thin and had short brown hair and a spunky cheerleader attitude. Over the last two years, both Lauren and Tatum had admitted that they suffered from eating disorders and had asked for our Bible study to pray for them. I had never seen them gain any weight. If anything, they continued to lose more pounds. Perhaps this is why neither of them had ever mentioned how fragile my body had become over the last year and a half. Instead, they told me repeatedly "how good" I looked. As I began to cry, Tatum put her arm around me. "Rach, we're here for you," she said. "We just want to make sure that the decision you made was what God wanted for you."

"Yes," Lauren jumped in. "We've been talking about this all week. We want to encourage you to search your heart to make sure this breakup is God's will for your life." I continued to cry softly, confused and lost.

They both put their arms around me. "We've been praying for you," said Tatum. "God has put it on our hearts to share this with you. We just feel like John is such a godly man, and it's normal for relationships to have bumps along the way. This is where your faith in God comes in!"

I sat silent as I listened to what they had to say. They talked at me for the next twenty minutes. Before I walked out of Lauren's apartment, they gave me big hugs and told me to pray and "listen to God."

All night I tossed and turned in bed, restless with questions that I couldn't answer. "Were my parents right? Was the timing just off? Did God choose John as my partner? Was I ignoring God? Did I lose my faith?" Some very small voice kept saying to me, "You did the right thing." Somewhere, in between all my questions and doubts and fears, my instincts were reassuring me, not of God or His "plan," but that I had made a safe decision for me.

I decided not to go back to Bible study the next week—or the week after that. No one called or texted me to ask why I didn't show up, which made me feel like I wasn't wanted back at the Bible study as a single woman. I felt like no one cared if I was okay. They only cared if I was following "God's plan" to be with John, which pushed me even farther away from ever returning. The church, the community that I had belonged to my whole life, seemed to ignore my heartache because my breakup didn't fall in line with what they believed as God's will for my life.

For the next two years, I saw these girls all over campus. They didn't ever acknowledge the fact that I never came back to their Bible study. We would make pleasantries, but the conversation never went beyond "Hi! Hope all is well!" In later years, I learned that John told Campus Crusade we had broken up because of my "lack of faith in God" and my "sexual desires that couldn't be controlled." I'm sure this is why Lauren or Tatum never asked me where I was or why I didn't come back to Bible study. They didn't want someone like me, living in sin, to be a part of their group. This separation quickly reminded me of the lesson I learned after I wore that beautiful hot pink dress to my first Cotillion, the night of my first assault: People are yearning to believe men and even more eager to doubt women.

Therapy

Even though Tatum, Lauren, and the other girls in my Bible study failed to recognize my current fractured state, my new resident assistant friends were very aware of my deepening depression and my continual weight loss. Hilary, with her small-town charm and kind heart, and Greta, an outspoken, independent brunette, both confronted me a few weeks after ending my engagement to John. They had noticed my evident eating disorder and my downward spiral of depression. A lot had changed since I met them a few months before in August. I had left my fiancé and the religious community. Everything I knew to be my world, John and my church community, had disappeared practically overnight. I felt lost. My plans for the future were no longer an option. So what would I do? What next?

I tried to bury the loneliness and despair through anorexia and bulimia, a two-sided disease that I had struggled with for years, even before John's emotional abuse started. Without the church, I felt strange, traumatized. The people who were my friends, who had walked on the path with me to become more like God, had now vanished. All I had left were the "sinners" and "lost souls" that the church had always warned me against. Now I would have to recreate my community out in the world.

One night, during our weekly *Glee* party, Greta had turned one of her beds into a couch with long purple body pillows against the wall to act like the back of a couch. During a commercial, Hilary asked how I was doing. It didn't feel like the normal, "Hey! How are you doing?" This seemed considered, a sympathetic, "How have you been feeling?" The care and concern in her voice shook my façade. She knew I had ended my engagement with John, but I hadn't told anyone about the Bible study group or that I was no longer attending Campus Crusade. My voice tightened as I opened up, explaining what had happened with my Bible study and expressing all my loneliness. This was the first time in my life that I didn't have a church or Christian community surrounding me. I had no clue what to do.

Hilary and Greta listened intently until I finished verbalizing what had been consuming my thoughts for the last few months. Greta handed me one of her fresh homemade lemon cupcakes, which made the whole room smell like lemon zest. With a kind smile, she said, "Have you thought about talking to someone?"

"You mean like a pastor?"

"No," she said. "Like a therapist. You've gotten so thin, and you just seem so sad all the time. We're worried about you."

"That may be really good, Rach," Hilary added. "You've been through a lot in the last few months." I wasn't sure what to say. The idea of a therapist was foreign to me. My parents had always said that Christians should see pastors for counsel over any type of therapist because therapists will promote secular ideas and just "give you meds you don't need" while a pastor will lead you through your troubles in the way of God. But I didn't have a pastor or a Christian mentor anymore, so maybe a therapist would be a good idea.

"Do you know anyone I can see?" I asked.

Looking back on this time, I feel so grateful that students' mental health is a priority at Indiana University. They have a huge staff of therapists ready to help any student in need at just twenty-five dollars per session. Greta saw one of the university therapists and recommended him to me. I didn't tell my parents that I made an appointment, knowing they would be upset that I went to a therapist over a pastor. If I told them, I would also need to explain that I didn't have a pastor anymore. I planned to use part of my monthly RA stipend to pay for the session. My parents wouldn't need to know about it.

I walked into the health center on a Tuesday morning right after my first lecture of the day. Terrified, I walked in and out of the building three times before I actually made it to the fourth floor where the mental health offices were located. Deep breath. I opened the door to the waiting area on the fourth floor. Before the door could even close behind me, a nice woman at the desk welcomed me to the clinic with a bright white smile. She handed me some paperwork that included the normal requests: address, phone number, medical history. But the second page included a type of survey that I hadn't seen before. It asked questions like, "Do you feel happy?" with a sliding scale of 1-5, one being "not at all" and five being "absolutely." I filled out the survey honestly without giving it much thought because I was eager to just make it through the actual appointment. As I handed the paperwork back to the nice woman with the bright smile, she informed me, "He'll be with you in about fifteen minutes."

As I sat alone in the office, I studied the random pamphlets on the table next to me. I read one about multiple personalities, one about depression, one about anxiety, and so on until my doctor called my name. He was probably in his late forties, with a clean-shaved head, thick black framed glasses, worn-in brown loafers, and an energy that immediately felt safe. I followed him from the waiting room down a long hallway to his office. He held the door open for me as I walked in.

The room was larger than I imagined and there was no fainting couch, which I expected, based on the movies I had seen where people went to see a therapist. Two of the four walls were lined floor-to-ceiling with bookshelves crammed full of academic books. He had only two chairs in the room and motioned me to where I should sit—an overstuffed brown leather chair with a gray blanket thrown over the back. We both sat down. "So, my name is Dr. Polis," he said. "Welcome to my office. Can I get you anything?"

"Nice to meet you. No, I'm good," I responded as I fidgeted with the blanket behind the chair.

"So what would you like to talk about today, Rachel?" he asked.

"Well, I'm just like, I don't know . . . really sad lately, and I just broke up with my fiancé, which sucks. So yeah, that's it. Also, I don't really know what to do here. I've only ever talked to pastors about my feelings. Seeing a therapist is kinda outside of my religion, so I don't know . . ."

He searched my face as I continued to fidget with the gray blanket. There was something about him that made me feel comfortable with him, even though I was uncomfortable in the situation.

"Well, Rachel," he started, as he crossed his right leg over his left. "It sounds like you've been dealing with a lot over the last few months. Let's start by discussing the survey you completed when you got here. Then let's talk a little more about what you just shared with me. How does that sound?"

He slowly went through the questions I had answered, never concluding anything or expressing any dissatisfaction with my answers. Instead, Dr. Polis thanked me for my honesty and re-assured me that I wasn't "damaged" or "broken," two words that the church and John had ingrained into my identity. It was a stark contrast from the pastor who I had seen the summer before in my pre-marriage therapy with John. Over the course of my session with Dr. Polis, I learned that he was a retired pastor, which gave me a sense of peace. It made me feel comfortable, knowing that he was a former church leader. At that time, it made me feel more secure, like I wasn't completely outside of the church.

When I began to discuss what had recently happened in my life, I felt free to voice my sadness and loneliness—two things I had never talked about with that much vulnerability to anyone until then. The one-hour session went so quickly that, before I knew it, Dr. Polis began wrapping up our time together. Leaning in with his hands held together on his lap and with compassion in his eyes, he said, "Rachel, I would like to see you again. I think that, from today, I can see that you are struggling with depression and disordered eating. I would really like to help you overcome these things. Would you allow me to work with you?" I looked him in the eye and nodded with tears in my own eyes. He was so earnest. His perception overwhelmed me. This was the first time someone had ever let me speak freely without any judgment. No one else had ever heard me, seen my wounds, and wanted to help me without shaming me. I didn't know support like this existed.

I saw Dr. Polis twice a month until I graduated from Indiana University two years later. I will always look back on my sessions with him with such gratitude, knowing he was instrumental in helping me acknowledge and then work through my eating disorder, depression, and anxiety. During the first year that we met, when my eating disorder was at the height of anorexia and bulimia, Dr. Polis helped me end this destructive cycle by having me work with a nutritionist twice a week until I entered recovery. Although, I still work with a therapist today to grow my self-confidence and self-love (because self-acceptance is an unending journey), Dr. Polis and my nutritionist were the catalysts to help me overcome my body dysmorphia and begin my journey of self-love.

While Dr. Polis worked with my thoughts and my mind, my nutritionist showed me the ways my body can work for me with proper fuel. Dr. Polis helped me work through my fears of becoming "fat" and of losing control, while my nutritionist taught me how good my body could feel when I had proper nutrition. I began to realize that I didn't have to live my life exhausted from self-hatred and self-sabotage. As I started to fuel my body with nutrition instead of withholding calories from myself, I developed appreciation for my body. I appreciated my body's ability to easily run five miles without feeling like I would pass out any second from lack of fuel. I appreciated my body's ability to wake up early feeling full of clarity, without a throbbing headache or a stomach screaming with pain begging me for food. Slowly, this appreciation drowned out the hatred. My body was no longer my enemy.

At this time, I was so crippled by my anxiety that I suffered from panic attacks multiple times a week. My depression grew so dark that I could rarely get out of bed to go to class. Dr. Polis helped me overcome my fear of antidepressants and anti-anxiety medication so I could begin to live my life again. During one of our sessions, he calmly explained to me, "Sometimes the body needs help to get back on track. This doesn't have to be something you do for the rest of your life. You take Advil when you have a headache. These medicines are no different."

Then he referred me to a psychiatrist for depression and anxiety medication. Although I still feared the religious consequences of taking these medications, I also knew that I could not academically afford to keep skipping multiple classes a week because of my depression and anxiety attacks. Even though seeing a therapist and taking medication were completely outside of my religion and what I had been taught to be "God honoring," I noticed how

Dr. Polis helped me feel better than any pastor or any church had ever helped me in the past. I realized I needed his help to survive.

In my time with Dr. Polis, our conversations focused on my eating disorder recovery and regaining my self-worth that had disappeared long ago, when the church had taught me the evils of my womanhood. During our sessions, he had to probe with a lot of questions or sit silently for minutes until I became so uncomfortable with the silence that I spoke my thoughts into existence. I had never spoken openly about my thoughts or feelings without shame or fear of sin, so speaking with him felt like speaking a foreign language. I learned and we practiced. I opened up to him slowly and never fully—still fearful that he might flip a switch and become like Linda or Pastor Tim, filled with judgment and hate.

Even though we discussed John, for example, I kept the conversation on a very superficial level, sharing only my sadness about the relationship ending and my uncertainty that anyone would ever love me. I never spoke to Dr. Polis about how John abused me physically and emotionally behind closed doors. It would take me many more years before I could recognize John's emotional abuse, fully admit it, and speak openly about it to anyone.

So, That's It?

In February of my sophomore year, Greta planned a trip for us to visit her brother at Miami University in Oxford, Ohio. Her brother, Alex, was a senior there and had invited us to come stay with him at his fraternity house. A bartender at the local campus bar, Alex had also promised Greta that he would be able to get us into the bar, even though we were both under twenty-one.

When Greta brought up the idea of this weekend adventure to me, I felt hesitant to go. Although I had distanced myself from my church community, I still believed in God and considered myself a Christian. As a Christian woman, I knew that both drinking and spending the night in a fraternity with men that were not my husband fell into the sin category. But ever since I left my Bible study and Campus Crusade for Christ, I began to question all the rules of Christianity, which I previously accepted and followed blindly. Everything felt upside down, almost like clinging to my Christian morals meant finishing a marathon walking backwards. I no longer invested myself in a community that made me feel shameful and repent for my decisions, so I had begun testing the waters. I wanted to really decide what I personally believed, and what did and did not make me feel guilty outside of the church community. With a little push, Greta convinced me to go to Miami of Ohio for the weekend.

"I promise we'll have fun," she said as she packed her pink duffle bag into her maroon sedan. "You need a break after everything that's happened over the last few months. You can let loose. I promise my brother will take care of us."

Throwing my black purse into her back seat, I hopped into the passenger side of her car. "Okay," I said. "Let's do this!" I was ready to test my freedom.

After a two-hour car ride filled with our favorite musical show tunes, we arrived at Miami University, which is always top on the list of the "Most Beautiful Colleges in America." Robert Frost even called Miami of Ohio, "the most beautiful campus that ever existed." As we made our way to Alex's frat house, we admired the historic architecture and the majestic trees, still resplendent in green foliage, a welcome change from what most of the Midwest looked like in winter. In comparison to the rest of the campus, Alex's frat house had peeling purple paint and broken windows, exactly what you might expect when a bunch of college dudes live in a house together. We parked the car on the street, grabbed our duffel bags, and I followed Greta into the house.

"Alex! WEEEEE'RRREEE HERE!" Greta screamed with excitement. One of Alex's frat brothers came out of the living room to the entryway of the house to greet us.

"Hey, ladies! Alex went to grab beer. He'll be back in a little, but I told him I would keep you company until he got back." This was the guy Mark told us went by "Turtle" because all his "brothers" thought he reminded them of Turtle from *Entourage*. He was short, probably around 5'7" with blonde hair and blue eyes.

Wearing khaki shorts and an old tank top jersey with the frat's letters on it, Turtle held a Natural Light beer in his hand—the epitome of a frat boy. With a big smile and oozing confidence, he welcomed us to grab a beer and join him on the ripped navy-blue couches in the living room.

Greta drank her beer and chatted with Turtle and Alex's other brothers while I sat back quietly holding my Natural Light, unsure if I should drink it. I felt dizzy with all the contradictions rolling around in my head. I had always been taught that drinking alcohol is against God's plan, but at the same time, I was no longer in the church. Can I be a Christian and still have a drink? I decided I could.

Alex came back to the house a little while after we got there. He gave Greta and me a hug, welcoming us to his "lovely abode." Joking, he looked at Turtle on the couch. "Good!" Alex said. "You didn't fuck either of them. My sister and her friends are off limits, remember?" They both laughed and toasted cold beers in the air.

After we drank a beer or two downstairs, Alex walked us up the broken, sticky, beer-stained stairs to his room where we were staying in two bunk beds. He stayed at his girlfriend's house for the weekend.

"Can you guys be ready in like thirty minutes?" Alex asked.

"Oh, TOTALLY!" I said, feeling more confidence from my two beers.

"Cool. You guys get ready. Then I'll take you to my bar," he said as he walked down the stairs to drink more cheap beer in the living room with the guys.

Greta and I helped each other put on makeup and do our hair, trying to make us look older than we were. As she helped me straighten my curls, she said, "You know Turtle kept looking at you downstairs."

"No, he didn't," I said with a giggle. "Wait, but did he?"

"Totally! I think you should dance with him at the bar tonight."

"I mean, he's really cute. I wouldn't be opposed."

"Girl! Come on. You need some excitement and someone to have some fun with! Just flirt a little and see where it goes."

We finished getting ready and then went downstairs to meet the boys and walk to the bar. I wore a new tight black long sleeve shirt with sequins on it (the only semi-sexy thing I owned), dark jeans, and black heels. Greta had on a cute black dress and flats. When we met the boys in the living room downstairs, I felt Turtle's eyes on me. Maybe Greta was right? Maybe he was into me? Even the thought of him taking an interest in me had my body on fire. I hadn't really thought about boys since breaking up with John five months before, so to be reminded of what it felt like when someone takes notice of you felt exhilarating.

On the walk over to the bar, Turtle walked next to me. "Where are you from?" he asked. "What are you studying? What do you want to do after school?" You know, the typical questions. As we chatted, I thought to myself, "Be cool, Rachel. Don't mention the engagement. Play the cool, girl. You got this." We innocently flirted, and it felt great. I couldn't remember the last time I had flirted with someone. I wanted this feeling to keep going.

We got to the bar around 10:00 p.m. Alex walked us right in the front door, and no one even asked for our IDs. He got Greta and me our first drinks, White Russians. "WOW!" I said to her as I sipped the sweet, creamy drink. "This tastes amazing! So much better than those beers!" (After the first taste, I had reluctantly forced the beer down. I wanted to feel cool. I wanted to feel like I fit in with the Greek life culture, which I had never entered as a freshman because John refused to allow me to join a "slutty sorority.")

She laughed and gave me a hug. "I told you! This is going to be fun!"

The bar was dark, the music was loud, and the free drinks were flowing. I spent the first half of our time with Greta in the corner, half dancing, half giggling from the alcohol. I didn't know where Turtle went, and I didn't feel a need to look for him. I danced, just enjoying the moment with my friend in total freedom until I felt a hand slip around my waist. Turning around, I saw Turtle. Drunk and happy, he pulled me close. "Come dance with me," he said.

We danced together for a few hours, only taking breaks to go get more White Russians at the bar. Drink by drink, my inhibition and control were quickly drowning. As we danced, his hands wrapped around my waist; his lips met my neck with desire. I had completely forgotten what it felt like to be desired—to have someone touch you and your body spark with electricity. My body craved his. I didn't feel any guilt about it.

"LAST CALL!" the bartender shouted, interrupting my euphoria. Greta quickly grabbed my hand as she told Turtle to go get us two more drinks while we went to the bathroom. In the bathroom, Greta confronted me. "Rach! I don't know what's happening out there, but he is INTO you!"

Fixing my smeared black eyeliner in the mirror while holding onto Greta's hand for balance, I admitted my drunk confession to her. "So, I kinda wanna have sex with him. Is that bad? Are you going to judge me?"

Squeezing my hand, she reassured me. "I would never judge you. I just want to make sure that you want this? You aren't too drunk?"

"No. I may be drunk, but I want this."

We walked out of the bathroom with our arms linked. The bar appeared almost empty. The bartender told us to hurry with our drinks. Alex and Turtle slammed shots, while Greta and I quickly drank our last White Russians for the night. Alex left the bar to walk back to his girlfriend's house, while Turtle, Greta, and I walked back to the frat house together. Greta walked in front of me and Turtle as we held hands and kissed the whole way home. As we walked up the stairs to Alex's room, Turtle asked me if I wanted to come to his room across the hallway. I nodded and followed his lead. Before he closed the door, I could hear Greta scream, "Don't do anything I wouldn't do!" Then she laughed as she went to bed in Alex's room alone.

The alcohol had made all my nerves disappear. I felt nothing but euphoria as he undressed me, kissing every inch of my body as he did. We lay on his bed, him on top of me as he moved his kisses from my neck to my belly to in between my legs. My body shuddered as his mouth made me climax. He crawled back up so his face met mine. "Is it cool if we have sex?" I smiled and nodded, and he rolled on a condom before putting himself inside of me. The act didn't last very long before we both allowed the sleepiness from the alcohol to set in and passed out.

When I woke up the next morning, I quietly, almost like a spy, got out of his bed and grabbed my clothes. Peaking my head into the hallway to make sure no one would see me, I quickly darted into Alex's room. I climbed into bed with Greta and told her all about what had happened.

"Well? Do you feel different?" she asked me curiously, knowing my previous virgin status.

Taking inventory of my body for the first time that morning, I looked at her with surprise. "Actually, no," I said.

The thing is, I felt the same as I had the day before. In fact, if anything, I felt better than the day before. I didn't feel like I had "lost a piece of myself," or like I was "damaged." I didn't feel like I was "bonded" to this guy. In fact, I didn't really expect to ever talk to him again, and I felt okay with that. I didn't find anything special or magical about what had happened. He made me feel good. I didn't feel any guilt or shame about that. But I kept asking myself, "So that's it?" Why had I believed I would feel horrible, overwhelming guilt and shame if I experienced sex outside of marriage? *My value is virginity. Sex outside of marriage will leave me alone.* Why had I always been taught that this act would change me? How did I feel more guilt and shame for only giving John a blowjob than having sex with a man I knew I would never see again? What could I be missing?

As I lay in bed contemplating these questions and replaying everything that I had experienced with John in comparison to what I had experienced the night before with Turtle, I began to realize that maybe my freedom to choose was why these experiences felt like polar opposites. I had chosen what I wanted, instead of God, my church, or John deciding what was good for me. My body felt more like my own than it had my entire life. I loved the feeling.

Flying Free

May quickly arrived, bringing my sophomore year at IU to an end. The gorgeous campus was fruitful with all the flowers in full bloom and all the trees finally filled with green leaves again. Mom and Dad decided that it would be beneficial for me to live with my widowed aunt in New York City for the summer, telling me that "she wanted help with her business" and "some companionship for the summer would be good for her."

They framed my summer visit to Aunt Frida's as a way I could help, but I knew they actually wanted her to help me, thinking a change of scenery may brighten my demeanor. They had seen my mental state during that winter and watched me change majors from pre-med to hospitality and tourism management because my depression caused me to miss too many organic chemistry and biology classes to pass the courses. So I chose to transfer to tourism management as the majority of my credits transferred over to this new major. I knew this worried them, even though they never verbalized their concerns. Regardless, I was excited to live with Aunt Frida that summer in Manhattan. I had dreaded spending all summer in Portage, Indiana, where it felt like everywhere I looked, vivid flashbacks of John and my failed engagement would occur.

Packing up my dorm room during finals week, I heard my phone ring. Looking down at the caller ID on my pink blackberry, the screen read, "incoming call from John." I sat on my bottom bunk with the vibrating phone in my hand, debating whether I should pick it up or not. We hadn't spoken since we broke up last fall. Although I missed him every day, I had refocused my energy on my new major and my new community of friends. The call had one more ring before it went to voicemail. I decided to pick it up.

"Hello?" I answered.

"Hey, Rach." His familiar voice sounded good to my ears. "It's me, John."

"Hey. I know. Um . . . what's up? I mean, why are you calling? Is everything okay?"

"Yes, I just wanted to ask if you would meet me for coffee before we leave for the summer. I have some stuff I want to talk to you about."

I sat silent for a moment, debating if I should meet him, but my curiosity got the best of me. "Okay," I said. "Sure."

We made plans to meet the next day at the Starbucks on campus. I spent the next twenty-four hours filled with anxiety about what might happen when we met. I had no idea what to expect or why he wanted to meet with me. I changed my outfit at least ten times that morning before deciding on a simple, classic look—white T-shirt, blue jeans, and sandals.

Walking into Starbucks, I immediately laid eyes on him. He was wearing cargo shorts and a preppy yellow button-down shirt that I had given him the year before on his birthday. He smiled at me as our eyes met. I missed that smile. Sitting down at the table he had saved for us, he then handed me a coffee.

"I got here early, so I ordered your coffee," he explained.

"Thank you." I took a sip before asking him why he wanted to meet with me.

"Well, over the last few months without you, I've been praying a lot and seeking God's plan for moving forward. I wanted to meet with you because God has put it on my heart that we are meant for each other—you and me."

I sat stunned. Coming to meet him, I didn't know what to expect, but it definitely wasn't this. He continued as I silently stared at him. "God meant for us to be together, Rachel. I tried to date other women, but God kept telling me 'No. Rachel is for you.' Can't you feel it? It's his plan for us."

"So, you want to get back together?" I interrupted as I sat processing everything.

He nodded. "Yes. I know you were unhappy with me before, but I've changed a lot. I really am living my life in total submission to God."

My face felt lifeless, like it had instantly received thirty units of Botox. "I'm going to be honest with you. This is all a lot, and I don't know what to think right now. Plus, I'm going to live with Aunt Frida in New York this summer."

"I get that. I'm going to be living in Chicago this summer, working as a missionary for Youth for Christ, but we need to figure out how we're going to move forward."

How we're going to move forward? I thought, as I stared at him expressionless, unable to speak or move my face.

"I'll be in Portage for the next two weeks before I leave for Chicago. Will you be in Portage before you leave for NYC?" he asked me.

"Yeah. I'm going to be home for about a week and a half."

"How about we talk more on Saturday when we both get back home? Then you can think on this, and we can decide how we'll move forward."

There it was again, how WE move forward.

We both stood up from the table. He wrapped his arms around me. His familiar body felt good against mine. "I've missed you so much. Haven't you missed me?" he asked earnestly.

I had missed him, like you always miss your first love. "Yes. I have," I told him, as I allowed my body to sink deeper into our embrace. In this moment, all the good memories flooded through my mind like a crystal-clear waterfall washing away all the dirty bad memories. It's true. I missed the idea of him. I missed the companionship. I missed the certainty of an engagement and marriage. I missed what I thought was love. I missed the community of the church.

For the next several days, as I packed up my dorm room and moved my stuff home to my parents' house for the summer, I kept asking myself, "Why did I break up with him?" I knew I wasn't happy at the end of our relationship, but was there something else I was missing? Was I happy now? I prayed all week asking God for a sign. Asking God if John was right. Asking God if John was the man he had prepared for me. Asking God to just fucking answer me. I prayed and prayed, but God never answered.

Even though I no longer attended church or Campus Crusade for Christ anymore, I still believed in God. I still called myself a Christian. I just had difficulty navigating it all without the community I had always been involved in. I tried to live a life that pleased God, but my evolving mindset overwhelmed me daily, making everything I once believed as fact oppose the new freedoms I came to appreciate. I constantly doubted my decisions, comparing and evaluating them to what the church taught me were sins, sins that may keep me from heaven. *The blessings of eternal life. The blessings of joy. The blessings of a godly husband.*

These "truths" no longer felt like absolute truths, though. They felt like bondage, which I slowly elected to break through. How could I enjoy my life and still love God? Was this possible? I didn't feel the shame or guilt the church told me I would feel from having sex, or drinking, or not attending church. Instead, I started to feel free, crawling to a newfound independence, which excited me. But can these two worlds live at peace together? Could I be a woman of God and a "sinner"?

That Saturday night, John came over to my parents so we could talk. Mom and Dad were so excited that John and I might be rekindling our relationship that they left the kitchen to give us alone space. They had a great relationship with him. They loved him, but even more than that, he fulfilled their most important requirement—A Christian Man.

Everyone in my life saw the side of John that he wanted

them to see—kind, driven, living his life 100 percent for God, honorable. No one saw the side of John that I had seen—angry, judgmental, and abusive (something I couldn't even reconcile or verbalize until years later). Which is why it proved so difficult for me to end the relationship and so easy for me to take him back. To everyone else, he was perfect. According to John and the girls in my Bible study, I had made a mistake. God disapproved of my decision.

John and I sat in my parents' red-and-white kitchen that night discussing what came next. He told me over and over again that God laid on his heart that we were "God's perfect match." Then he asked me, "Don't you want to honor God?" I *did* want to honor God. That's all I had wanted since I sat in church as a little girl. I wanted to live a blessed life that led me to heaven. Maybe John was right. I had been disobedient to God by breaking up with him. Okay. He was probably right. I had left the church and been living a life of sin. How could I know what God wanted when I hadn't given him my all? *God is everything. I am nothing.*

"I want you to know that . . . I forgive you for leaving me and disobeying God's plan for our lives," he told me as he held my hand at the kitchen table. "I forgive you because God told me to."

Within a few hours he had turned this into a "me" issue. I wasn't honoring God. I was disobedient. I was wrong. I was ungodly. And I believed him. Within those few hours, he had me crying and begging his forgiveness. I went back to my abuser, as

I've now learned too many abused women do. If God's plan were for us to be together, then I would follow his plan.

After I had asked for John's forgiveness and said that I would get back together with him, he moved his chair closer to mine. "There's something else God has told me. He told me that you have sexually sinned with another man. I can't forgive you completely until you admit this to me."

I started crying again, all the shame and guilt I had hidden away after my experience with Turtle came running through my body like the cold rush of an IV fluid through my veins. "I don't know what to say. I um . . . I did have . . . I did have sex with another guy." Since I hadn't been in the church community for a while, I hadn't really felt any deep shame or guilt over this. I made my own decision that night. I wanted it to happen, and it felt good.

Looking at me with anger in his eyes, he said, "I think that it's going to take me awhile to forgive you for this." He stood up. Towering over me and looking down at my submissive body, he said, "I wanted to marry a virgin. Now that's gone. You gave it away, for what?"

Still crying, I whispered, "I'm sorry . . . I'm so sorry," as my body caved into itself in deeper submission.

"I need you to prove to me that I'm your only one. Are your parents in bed?" he asked.

I nodded as he stood over me and grabbed my hand. He led me

to my bedroom where I was once again on my knees for him—to prove my love and commitment. Afterwards, he made me pray like he had so many other times, but this time, he made me pray that God would forgive my sexual sin and that God would "show His mercy" to make me a "renewed virgin."

Within just one night, I came back. I belonged to him again. The role I had played and rehearsed for three years with John came back to me instantly— almost like the lines I rehearsed to play Emily and can still recite ten years later . . . both roles seemed to be a part of me that I could not break. He manipulated me so quickly this time. So quickly, I went from healing to becoming a ghost again. I wasn't doing anything for myself. I allowed the situation to happen to me.

A lot of strange things come with abuse, but one thing consistently stands out to me as I look back on this time in my life. For abuse victims, it's easier to believe your abuser telling you that it's your fault because believing that it's your fault means you have control.

John and I dated long distance all summer. He worked as a missionary for Campus Crusade in Chicago, while I worked for my aunt in NYC. We Skyped almost every day to talk about what we had been up to, and so he could lead us in prayers. The calls were innocent. It felt nice to have a familiar love in my life again, until our last call at the end of the summer. This call was different from all the others because this was the call he made to tell me that he had fallen in love with a girl who he worked with on his mission trip. "God told me to fall in love with her," he said. I sat shocked. "God led us to each other," he explained, "because she's pure. He is blessing me with a virgin because of my obedience to Him." Again, I sat frozen, unable to speak.

I didn't eat for days after John's call. What I did try to eat, I couldn't keep down. These were the darkest few weeks of my life. The five months of sessions I spent with Dr. Polis and everything we worked toward felt undone. I felt worthless. I thought no man would ever want me. John was right, and this time he had broken my spirit completely. The only good thing about this breakup was that when people asked what had happened and I told them that he cheated, they were on my side. I had something concrete to share with Dr. Polis when I returned to school in the fall. Being cheated on explained my tears and heartbreak. Telling my friends and family that John cheated seemed much more acceptable than just telling them that "I wasn't happy" or actually diving into the reality of the abuse I had endured.

The heart is a magical thing. It can so easily be shattered, causing a person to become lifeless, but no matter what the heart endures, it always heals with time. A few months after John cheated, my heart began to heal. I worked with Dr. Polis and slowly began piecing myself together. During the winter of my junior year, I decided to visit a tattoo shop with my close friend Hilary. I desperately wanted to cover up the matching tattoo that John and I had gotten two years ago, the summer before we went to IU together. This tattoo was the last reminder of his existence in my life.

As I sat in the chair, the artist looked at the cross tattoo on my left foot, inspecting it to see how he could cover it up. "It's going to need to be pretty big and all black," he said. "What did you have in mind?"

Hilary gave my hand a supportive squeeze as I sat in the big, black leather tattoo chair, confidently saying to the tattoo artist, "A bird . . . a bird flying free. I want her to soar."

When he finished, she looked beautiful, her wings flying with endless potential.

The Little Black Book

My junior year at IU became my year of rebuilding. At this point, I understood that I could not be a member of that church or of Campus Crusade for Christ. I also knew that John would never again be part of my life. The church didn't want me as a single woman living outside of "God's plan" of marriage to John. They also didn't want me as a sinful woman who spoiled her virginity. Everything I had thought would change after the summer, having John in my life again and reentering my Christian community, were no longer options. I had to come face to face with that fact.

To leave the church meant that I accepted the fate of Hell.

It meant that either I believed in God and accepted Hell, or I rejected God and Christianity, believing in nothing. Both options terrified me to my core. Some days were good. Most days I felt so convinced that I would end up in Hell, that I fell into a deep depression and self-hatred. I couldn't even get out of bed. Daily I had to combat the loud voice in my mind telling me I was unworthy of love or happiness—that I was useless. Some days I screamed at the voice, telling him, "THERE IS NO HELL," but most days the voice screamed at me: YOU ARE WORTHLESS. YOU ARE A SINNER. YOU BELONG IN HELL.

I almost lost my job as an RA because I became too shattered to care for the needs of my residents. I had to drop several classes because I couldn't break my bedridden depression to attend lectures. Dr. Polis and I worked together every week. I know that it's because of him that I never got to a place of self-harm, even when I had dark thoughts. Still, there was so much of me that needed to be put back together.

Midterm season came quickly. I needed several high scores to boost my GPA from failing almost all my organic chemistry and biology exams the year prior. I knew I couldn't trust myself to study in my dorm room because I would just fall asleep or watch TV, so I decided to go to the library stacks for a few dedicated study hours. The stacks at the IU library were ten floors of rows and rows and rows of books. Quiet and normally desolate, the stacks were the perfect place to cram for my exams. I arrived and picked a random, dismal floor, where I found an empty desk and began to study. After a few hours of cramming with flash cards and rereading my notes, I decided to take a break and walk through the stacks.

Walking through aisles and aisles of books, passing by thousands of titles, one title specifically caught my attention—a black book with a simple, small white font that read *The Purity Myth* by Jessica Valenti. Intrigued, I picked up the book and read the back cover: "A brave call to overhaul the way America measures young women's worth, *The Purity Myth* calls on all of us to put an end to the dangerous burden that falls on our girls to conform to the impossible standards of purity."

Curious, I decided to check out the book and read more in my dorm room that night. Over the next week, I carefully read every word that Valenti had written. *The Cult of Virginity. Classroom Chastity, Sex, Morals, and Trusting Women.* Page by page, chapter by chapter, I felt like Valenti spoke directly to me. In this book, she delicately unpacked the harm that the virginity movement inflicts on young women. Valenti detailed how the church uses sex and sexuality to control women, and then how they use this control in an attempt to keep women in traditional gender roles—wife, mother, and caretaker.

Everything Valenti wrote resonated with my soul. I remembered the little red book my mother gave me, the bullying I had experienced at the hands of men at Christian school, and the pre-marriage counseling I had attended with John. I read on as Valenti explained how toxic purity balls are. The idea that a young woman would pledge her purity to her father until he gives it to another man is ownership of a woman by one man until that man decides another man can own the woman's purity. She explained how damaging it is that morality within Christianity focuses on keeping a woman's hymen intact, instead of discussing morality as compassion, kindness, courage, and integrity. She dove into the idea that virginity is singularly a woman's pursuit—that women must be pure in order to be desired, but that men's value is not placed on their purity. *My value is virginity. Sex outside of marriage will leave me living alone.* I kept reading as Valenti tackled the fact that the purity movement within Christianity completely negates the natural sexual desire that all women feel because in fundamentalist Christianity, it's unnatural for women to have sexual desire and sexual pleasure. Her direct words and use of language sang to my soul, responding to all the questions and doubts I felt for years regarding religion and my sexuality.

As I read, I remembered myself as a little girl, with wild red curls sitting on my bottom bunk bed in Albany, Georgia, reading the Christian books my parents had given me on sexuality, purity, and becoming a God-fearing woman. Something clicked. I had lived my life being told what to do, how to live, and how shameful I should feel. The church and my family had taught me what part I needed to play in order to become a godly woman worthy of love and God's perfect plan. Until this point, I had played that role to perfection. Now as I read Valenti's book, I realized who I wanted to be. It was not anything that anyone had taught me or the church had forced upon me. The role was me—unapologetically and freely me. But who was I without the church and without John?

After finishing *The Purity Myth*, I craved more books like it. I had never read any nonfiction, non-Christian books, so after acing my finals and before heading back to Portage for winter break, I decided to ask my friend Jessie for suggestions. Jessie, a loud and proud feminist, worked with me at the dorm part time. She had short red hair and a tattoo that read FEMINIST on her ribs. In addition to working with me at the dorm, she also volunteered for Planned Parenthood and the campus sexual assault prevention group. I knew she'd have reading suggestions for me—and she did!

I started with *She Comes First: The Thinking Man's Guide to Pleasuring a Woman*, reading it with wild fascination. Book after book, I began to realize that things I once felt so much guilt and shame for were actually normal! My sexuality was not sinful. I wasn't broken. I wasn't worthless. I was normal. My sexual desire is normal.

RECOVERY

what is the greatest lesson a woman can learn

that since day one
she's already had everything she needs within herself
it's the world that convinced her she did not

    – Rupi Kaur, The Sun and Her Flowers

Evangelical CrossFit

During Thanksgiving of my senior year at Indiana University, I went on my first trip to Denver. My friend Holly invited me to stay with her over the holiday weekend. I excitedly accepted the invitation. When I landed on the Tuesday evening before Thanksgiving, I quickly jumped in a cab to meet Holly at her apartment downtown. I will never forget seeing the mountains for the first time. To me, they looked surreal—like a painting you might find in an art museum, an untouchable beauty, but somehow within reach. After my short cab ride, I quickly arrived at Holly's downtown apartment, a place that looked like a dream—stunning, with light granite counter tops, dark wood cabinets, light wood floors, and beautiful coordinating furniture.

"So this is it!" Holly said, as she motioned to her living room and kitchen.

"Wow! This is beautiful!" I said, realizing that this apartment, although only a one bedroom in comparison to my parents' four-bedroom house, was aesthetically as nice as my parents' home in Indiana. I thought you had to be well into middle age before having such a nice home. I was inspired that Holly, at twenty-eight, could easily afford a luxury apartment like this one.

"Thanks, Rachel!" Holly responded, plopping down on her gray sectional couch. Then she began combing through her shiny blonde hair. "Are you hungry?" she asked me. "I already ate, but if you're hungry, you should walk over to Linger."

Linger, Holly explained, was a hot new restaurant in Denver, a fifteen-minute walk from her apartment. She suggested that I grab dinner there while she finished up some work emails. I took her directions and walked over to the restaurant. A pretty hostess welcomed me, asking if I'd like to sit inside or on the rooftop bar.

"Well, does the rooftop have good views?" I asked.

"Oh—the best views in the city. You can see the skyline and the mountains."

"Upstairs, it is then! Thank you!"

The hostess then led me up a black metal winding staircase to the rooftop. When we reached the rooftop, I noticed the bright vintage décor surrounding the mid-century modern tables and chairs. Next to the seating area, a light teal vintage Volkswagen van, which had been gutted, was being used as a rooftop bar. This was WAY cooler than any restaurant I had ever been to in Indiana or Chicago.

I will never forget sitting on the Linger rooftop drinking their homemade red sangria while studying the view of the city in front of me, with a wide landscape of unending mountains to my right. The city skyline glittered under the stars, highlighting the curves and ridges of the mountains against the moonlight. I sat intoxicated by the beauty of this city. In that moment, I felt okay. My heart was not healed by any means, but right then, I knew I would heal. I felt it in the mountain breeze. I knew that I would heal in this city. There were possibilities for me here. This city was exactly where I needed to be after graduation.

My final months at Indiana University came and went quickly. Before I knew it, I was walking across the stage to receive my diploma in Hospitality and Tourism Management and then packing for my move to Denver. Mom and Dad came down to Bloomington, Indiana, about three-and-a-half hours southeast of Portage, to celebrate my cum laude graduation and help me get ready for my move to Denver. They were very proud of my cum laude distinction, telling all their friends and all our family about my accomplishment. Even though they didn't say it, I felt how proud they were of my survival through my depression. I could see the emotions in my parents' eyes, even if their emotions went unsaid.

Luckily, my parents understood about children leaving their families in pursuit of their dreams. My mom had moved from her small farming town (of less than 300 residents) in upstate New York to New York City after college. My dad had joined the military after college. We had also moved so much as a family that my move seemed almost unsurprisingly minor to Mom and Dad. I remember telling them, a few months before, that I had decided to move to Denver. Mom seemed sad but also hopeful for my new life, reminiscing with me about her journey after college and how she had ultimately created her own beautiful life.

Dad didn't say much as Mom rambled through her hopes and dreams for me. Finally, Dad interrupted. "You know what, Rach? Take the chance! If you don't like it, you can move home. What's the worst that could happen?" Although, they were sad that we wouldn't be able to see each other often, my parents understood the importance of branching outside your family and comfort zone in order to make a home for yourself. By leaving their own homes, they had met and started their own love story.

As we packed, I will never forget how Mom grabbed my hand, looked me in the eyes, and told me with such earnest belief, "This is what we have prepared you for. Go stretch your wings and fly." Mom and Dad had no idea that I no longer attended church or Campus Crusade, as I frequently lied and told them how both communities were "challenging me" and "growing my love for God daily." Lying seemed easier then breaking their hearts, so I chose the lie as their deliverance. When we were together, I played the part of their godly Christian daughter. They thought nothing had changed . . . even though everything had changed. I played my role well, so they had no hesitation about my move to Denver. In their minds, if I survived four years at IU and came out of a liberal college as a godly Christian woman, Denver could never cause me to lose my faith.

In May of 2013, Dad drove his black Honda CRV, and I drove my black Kia Optima, a gift from Nana after she could no longer drive, fifteen hours from Indiana to Colorado. To this day, the move is one of my proudest accomplishments. I decided what I wanted my life to look like, and I took the risk of moving fifteen hours from home with no job and only one friend, Holly, who assured me that she would be my guide through this new city of mine. During the long drive, I felt many conflicting emotions: fear, excitement, doubt, belief, and longing, but in all these emotions, I felt certain that Denver was the right place for my new journey. Dad and I arrived at my new apartment off of Speer Boulevard in the Golden Triangle neighborhood around 10:00 p.m. My simple apartment with its laminate wood floors, white walls, and green kitchen countertops made me feel at peace the minute I walked in.

The next morning, Dad took me to American Furniture Warehouse to buy me a new mattress before he started the drive back home. We tried out about twenty mattresses before I picked my mattress: a firm, full-size mattress on sale. Dad wanted to buy me the box spring too, but I wouldn't let him. He had already taken several days off of work to make this journey with me and had helped me pack and unpack all my stuff. A $300 mattress seemed more than generous in my mind. On our way home from the mattress store, I asked him if we could stop at Brother's Bar in downtown Denver. Brother's Bar, a chain sports bar, is where I waitressed during my senior year at IU. I hoped that this location would hire me until I could find a career job. While Dad waited in the car, I walked in with confidence. Then, fifteen minutes later, I walked out with a job and three shifts that week. Dad high-fived me after I jumped into the black CRV and told him I got the job. "You see, Rach," he said, "This is what Overvolls are made of—will and determination! We don't let anything stop us when we put our minds to something."

Before Dad had to begin his drive back to Indiana that afternoon, we grabbed burgers at Highland Tap and Burger. Dad, with his cleanly shaved bald head, khaki pants, and brown straw fedora, and me, with my long, straightened red hair and white jean shorts, sat on the patio talking for hours, stretching out our final time together. We both knew it would be a few months before we saw each other again. When our visit ended, I looked at him and thanked him for all his help with my move and for all his support.

Fidgeting with his fork, picking up the final crumbs of French fries on his plate, Dad looked at me with tears in his eyes. "I'm so proud of you Rach. You decided what you wanted, and you went for it. You have so much courage." This was the first time I really felt my father's acceptance of my adulthood. My dad no longer stood above me with judgment or watched my every move, waiting to provide godly correction. He looked at me with pride at the person I had become, the person he helped to shape. We stood up and hugged for a long time before he got into his CRV and started the fifteen-hour drive back to Portage. As I watched his car drive away, a realization took my breath away, like a ball to the chest in a dodgeball match—I was really here. I was really alone.

The next morning was Sunday. Although I had promised my parents that I would find and attend a church that morning, I decided that I would much rather attend the free morning workout at the Lululemon in Cherry Creek. Denver is a well-known fitness city, so I knew that this class would be a great opportunity to meet some new people. I arrived at the store in all the Lululemon I owned at that time—a baby pink tank top and black Capri leggings. The tank top, a final sale item, had been a birthday gift from my mom. I had bought the leggings online a few months before. At $128 for one pair of leggings, these were definitely the most expensive piece of clothing I had ever bought for myself, making me feel like a real member of the Lulu club when I walked into the store. Feeling proud but anxious to meet people, I entered the store and discovered that a local CrossFit gym was sponsoring this weekend's free workout. I had never lifted a weight in my life. The majority of my workouts for the last two years had revolved around training for half marathons. I immediately felt pretty intimidated by all the abs and muscles in the white showroom.

Standing in the back as the gym owner welcomed us, I saw Rick, a short, muscular man in his mid-thirties with dark hair, facial scruff, and a backwards "CrossFit" hat. He walked us outside to the stations in front of Lululemon. One by one, he explained what we would be doing for one minute at each station—rowing, box jumps, kettlebell swings, and overhead press. Rick stood on top of a tan wood box as he enthusiastically finished the instructions: "Everyone find a partner, and LET'S GO!" As people quickly paired off with their friends, I looked around and made eye contact with a tall, tan woman wearing black Lululemon shorts and a sports bra that showed off her toned six-pack. She made friendly eye contact back, walking over to me to introduce herself. "Hi! I'm Christine. Want to be partners?"

Relieved that I wasn't the last person standing, something that happened all throughout high school gym class, I smiled. "Sure thing!" I said. "I'm Rachel!"

We chitchatted for a few minutes before the workout began. Christine asked me if I had done CrossFit before. I explained that I hadn't, but I had just moved to town and wanted to socialize. "Well, this is a great way to meet people," she said, as she bent down to re-tie her purple Reebok sneakers. "Let's talk more after the workout."

"3-2-1. GO!" Rick yelled as we began our first minute sprint of kettlebell swings. I felt breathless quickly. I was still getting acclimated to the altitude and had never before engaged in such an intense workout. At each station, Christine, Rick, and some of the other gym members encouraged me on. Their support reminded me of the thrill and adrenaline rush I always felt before crossing the finish line at one of my races, using the cheers of the crowd to propel my final steps.

When we finished our workout, we all high-fived each other before I collapsed on the sidewalk to gulp down my water. Christine and Rick came over and sat next to me. "You did great today!" Rick said, as he gave me another high five. "Rachel, right?"

"Yeah! Thanks," I replied, still out of breath. "I was pretty nervous. I'm more of a runner, so this was new for me."

"Totally! Christine told me you're new to town? You should come by the gym this week! We have a great community and lots of people for you to meet."

"Yeah, girl! Come by!" Christine added. "It'll be awesome!"

I agreed and made plans to come to a class the following Saturday morning. During the week, I applied for jobs during the day and worked my three shifts at Brother's Bar at night. All week, though, my mind excitedly counted down the days until I could go to the gym and meet more people. I needed a lively, supportive community. According to Rick and Christine, this was what the CrossFit gym offered. I remember looking forward to that class like I looked forward to church services as a little girl. Saturday morning came, and Rick and Christine welcomed me along with some other new faces. The workout again made me feel as if I were on the verge of fainting. I didn't really like it, but I liked the people I had met and the acceptance I felt, so when Rick asked me after class if I wanted to become a member of the gym, I exuberantly said yes.

For the next three years, I went to the CrossFit gym at least five days a week. When I wasn't in the gym, I talked about the gym to anyone who would listen and spent all my time outside of work with people from the gym. Every weekend I worked out in the morning or watched other members of the gym workout at CrossFit competitions. Then I went to a bar with gym members or to a gym member's house to drink for the night. I ate a Paleo diet (basically no grains or sugar), baked Paleo desserts, and obsessed over gaining muscle and losing weight. Growing up, I was completely consumed by the church and the community the church provided for my family. I think on some level, it seemed natural for me to leave one community only to become consumed by another. Except, instead of preaching the gospel of Christ, I preached the gospel of CrossFit.

Although the CrossFit community can be very welcoming, the community itself is highly competitive, which did not fare well for my eating disorder recovery. Being in constant competition with others made me feel meaningless. As much as I went to the gym and trained for hours every week, my workout was never the fastest, my weights were never as heavy as the other women, and my body was never as muscular. As with church, I tried to be the best, but I never seemed to be able to get there. So I obsessed over my failures. I continued to live in the "I am worthless" mindset even away from the church. *God is everything. I am nothing. CrossFit is everything. I'm not good enough.*

I couldn't see it then but being invested in a body-focused community became toxic for my eating disorder recovery. The competitive mindset of the community and the rigorous mental and physical workouts pushed me into a constant battle with my body. I wasn't binging and purging anymore, but I did limit my calorie intake severely, cutting out a major nutrient source (hello, carbs!) in order to adhere to the Paleo diet. My food restrictions and over-exercise became especially intense a few months before I took a vacation to Mexico with a group of friends from the gym.

The Mexico vacation came about a year and a half after starting my CrossFit "journey." I began working in customer service for a luxury hospitality company. As part of our work perks, we could take two complimentary vacations per year at one of the company's luxury houses around the world. To celebrate my 24th birthday, I chose to go to Punta Mita, Mexico with a group of friends from the CrossFit gym. We started planning the June vacation a few months before, and, of course, a central topic of our conversations became how much we were going to work out so we would all look "hot."

Two of the women—April, a short, muscular woman with light brown hair and a teal nose ring, and Sophie, also incredibly muscular with dark shiny brown hair—and I kept each other accountable during the months before the vacation to eat strictly Paleo and to be in the gym as much as possible. It reminded me of high school days when my friends and I made sure we said our daily prayers. Keeping April and Sophie accountable seemed silly to me. They didn't even need to worry about their bodies being "beach ready." They both had six packs and toned arms already. However, their need to look better fueled my own insecurities and hatred of my body.

I looked nothing like them. I weighed about twenty pounds more than I had at the height of my eating disorder four years before. although I wasn't out of shape, I did not have six pack abs to show off like they did. For those two months before we left, I worked my ass off in the gym, severely limiting my calories so I would look like the people in my community.

June came, and before I knew it, April, Sophie, I and a few other gym friends were sipping cheap tequila on a plane heading to Mexico. When we arrived at our luxury beachfront villa, we all stood in awe. We could smell the saltwater of the ocean from our place. Our concierge took us on a tour of the 5,000 square foot villa. We admired the pure white floor tile, kitchen counters, and bathroom counters, which were accented with a décor of bright green and turquoise blue. As soon as our concierge finished the tour of the two-story villa, private pool, and large breakfast patio, we all rushed to put on our swimsuits and hit the beach below. To reward ourselves for all our hard work back home, April, Sophie and I had purchased Brazilian cut bathing suits—basically thongs and tiny tops. As we all walked down to the beach together in our new swimwear, I looked at my stomach and felt confident for all the work I had been putting into my body. I almost looked like them.

After playing in the ocean, drinking margaritas, and making sandcastles, the ladies decided to take a sunset picture showcasing our asses in our new Brazilian swimwear. Rick, who had first introduced me to the gym community, gladly took the picture for us. We stood with our arms around each other, backs facing the camera, with the clear blue ocean and bright pink sunset in front of us. I stood in the middle with blue bottoms and yellow bikini strings across my back, my red hair wavy from the salt water. Sophie stood to my left with her hot pink suit. April stood at my right in her bright green suit with her arm on my shoulder. We smiled with accomplishment, basking in our beach bodies during this impromptu photo shoot. As soon as Rick handed us back our iPhone with the picture, we all quickly posted it on Facebook and Instagram—ready to show off all our hard work! For the rest of the night, without any care in the world, we drank margaritas and laughed with our toes in the water.

When I work up the next morning on my 24th birthday, I immediately went to Facebook and Instagram to check out my "likes" and "comments" on my new picture. Opening the Facebook app to check my notifications, I saw the first one: "Aaron has tagged you in his status."

"Weird," I thought. Aaron was a guy from the CrossFit gym who I had briefly dated a few months before. By briefly, I mean really briefly—two or three dates. About a month before the trip to Mexico, we had gone to a bar with a group of people from the gym, and I had started dancing with another guy. Aaron and I weren't exclusively together, so I saw no problem with it. Someone else had asked me to dance, and I said yes. Aaron, however, saw a big problem with this. Although we had both made it clear that we were also dating other people, he did not approve of me dancing with another guy in front of him. The next day, he sent me a series of text messages, where he called me a "slut" and an "attention whore." I wasn't really hurt by the text messages. I had been called worse before by John, so I just brushed the texts off as "Aaron is crazy possessive. Good thing I learned that now. Time to move on."

So you can imagine my surprise, when I looked on Facebook to see that he tagged me in his status months after his demeaning texts. Lying in my bed in the crisp white room with turquoise-and-light-green decorations, I clicked the notification on my iPhone.

"Some girls should never post pictures in bikinis. It's like a train wreck that you can't unsee. @Rachel Overvoll."

"Holy shit! What the actual FUCK?" I remember thinking. This had to be a mistake. Why would he write something like this about me, someone he dated for less than two weeks? Jumping out of bed, I threw on my bathing suit from the day before. But this time, with a black dress over my suit, I ran upstairs to meet everyone for breakfast on our patio. Before I could even bring it up over our coffee and French toast, April and Sophie asked me about it.

"Um . . . so I saw Aaron's post on Facebook," Sophie said.

"Yeah, uhh, what do you think you did to make him so mad?" April asked, adding more coffee to her cup.

"I mean. I guess it was what happened last month? But like, how the fuck can someone be that cruel?" I replied.

For the rest of the day, I remember being outraged and feeling humiliated—and disgusting. I was infuriated that he felt okay to speak about someone that way—that he would post something like that on social media for everyone to see. The next five days in Mexico were mostly a blur. I drank too many margaritas and cried a lot. My friends were supportive, but my heart felt so hurt that none of their words seemed able to lift my spirit. It was like all the work I had done on myself to recover from my eating disorder came undone with sixteen words.

I thought I had overcome my indoctrination of believing that what men think of me was more important than what I thought of myself, but my reaction to his status proved otherwise. I purged a few times during the rest of the week and several times for the next few weeks—something I hadn't done in over two years. In that one post, Aaron had made all my internal self-hate and self-doubt seem true. I had spent years telling myself that I was "fat," "worthless," and "ugly," and, through recovery, had been trying to dig myself out of that hole. When someone comes along and tells you that what you have been telling yourself for so long is true, the hole feels too deep to ever get out.

When we got back from Mexico, I slowly stopped going to the gym. I went from going to five plus classes per week to attending one every week or every other week, until finally, I wasn't going at all. I felt the need to leave—just like what I did with the church. In order to make it official, I called up Mike, the gym owner. "Hey Mike. I need to cancel my membership," I told him as I lay on my bed at home. "I haven't been coming to the gym for a while. It just doesn't make sense anymore to pay if I'm not using the membership."

"Yeah, I've noticed that you haven't been coming. Does this have to do with what Aaron said? You know I told him he couldn't say those things to people in our community."

"Um, well, kind of. I just don't feel comfortable being around him. I feel like he stole some safety I felt in the community."

With confidence in his voice, Mike responded, "Come on, Rach. You just have to be the bigger person. Show up and show him you don't care."

I responded with a tight voice, trying to act like Mike's passive response didn't affect me. "I just think I need a break. Can you cancel my membership please?"

After that call, I lay in bed, immersed in a sense of déjà vu. This interaction seemed eerily similar to when I left the church. Both communities expected me to "be the bigger person" and "make it work" instead of calling the men involved out on their actions—100 percent accountability for women and 0 percent accountability for men. Mike told me he would freeze my account for "when I was ready to come back." I knew that I would never be ready to come back. Three years later, my account is probably still frozen. I wonder if my Campus Crusade for Christ membership is still frozen, too.

As the weeks went by, I began to realize that I didn't actually miss CrossFit at all. I missed the community, but the workouts and the Paleo diet? Nope, I didn't miss those one bit. When I left the church, I felt pretty much the same way. I missed the community; I didn't miss the rituals and services or the constant shame blanket I wore. Week by week, month by month, I began to rediscover my joy for running outside and the happiness that other new activities brought to my life. In fact, running became my church—it is where I go when I need to scream with joy or cry with sorrow. Running is how and where I discovered me.

During those months after CrossFit, I also learned that I loved yoga, barre, and hiking! Giving myself permission to try new experiences allowed me to learn what I actually enjoyed doing, which slowly began to bring my confidence back. With all the new activities I tried, I came to realize that I can be part of many communities. I didn't need to find one thing and obsess over becoming perfect at that one thing in order to build a community or feel happy. By slowly immersing myself in activities that brought me joy and freedom, I established myself in many communities and found my own chosen families.

Dating Daze

Now that I was no longer in the church, I didn't have to "court." I was finally able to freely date whoever I wanted, and in the manner I chose, regardless of religious affiliation or my parents' approval. But what dating habits should I choose? How do I even start dating? I felt as lost as a toddler in a corn maze, so I did what

I saw my friends were doing—I joined a couple of dating apps. First I created a profile on Tinder, then I copied that profile to Bumble, and within less than an hour of relaxing on the brown leather couch in my apartment living room, I opened myself up to the romantic possibility of thousands of men in Denver.

My profile picture was one of me and Daisy, my lab mutt rescue dog. In the picture, I was kneeling next to Daisy at the CrossFit gym, wearing a floral sports bra, tight black Nike shorts, and a big smile. I thought it was the perfect picture to showcase my interests—working out and my dog. At first, I remember being terrified to swipe right (for interested) or left (not interested) on the apps. Although I was no longer "sinning" by dating, something about the concept of meeting men on an app seemed dangerous or wrong. But after a few weeks of opening, then quickly closing the apps, I finally took the advice of my girlfriends and began swiping.

My first date was with Beau. Beau was a video editor and had just returned to Denver after spending his summer in Canada filming and editing a documentary about Iron Man athletes. He had long brown hair that touched his shoulders, with curls that hung in tight ringlets framing his blue eyes against tanned skin. We chatted for a few days on Tinder before deciding to meet in person at Denver Beer Co. Since Denver Beer Co. allows dogs, Beau had suggested this date spot so that I could bring along Daisy.

I remember getting ready that night for my first real date outside of religious expectations or my parents' standards. I could control what happened on the date and after. As I slipped on my white tank top and light blue jeans, I felt more freedom than nerves. Walking into the bar with Daisy a few minutes late, I immediately recognized Beau from his pictures. He was sitting at the bar with his curly hair pulled into a low bun. His blue eyes met mine with a welcoming smile. He stood up to hug me and before sitting back down in his seat, asked me what I'd like to drink.

"Um, a Princess Yum Yum please," I said. I wasn't much of a beer drinker, but I didn't want to tell him that, so I ordered the fruitiest beer on the menu in hopes the beer taste wouldn't overwhelm my pallet.

"A Princess Yum Yum it is!" he said with a kind smile.

The bartender quickly brought over our beers. Before he could give them to us, Beau and I had already found ourselves deep in conversation. For the next four hours, we sat at the bar engrossed with each other, talking about politics, travel, college, and life plans. The conversation flowed freely and with natural flirtation. Finally, at 10:00 p.m., I saw the bartender cleaning up the last table in the bar and realized how long Beau and I had been talking. It was as if we had been the only people in the bar. For the last four hours our attention had been solely focused on each other.

"Well, I think we're getting kicked out of here," I said to Beau with a grin.

"Yeah. I didn't really expect to close a bar down on our first date. Let me walk you home."

As we began our walk home with Daisy, Beau took my hand. "So what made you try this Tinder dating stuff?" he asked.

"Oh, you know," I said coyly. "It just seemed like the right time."

"Come on," he probed. "There has to be a story of a crazy ex-boyfriend or a heartbreak or something?"

I paused. The memory of John's face, his touch, my heartbreak, it all rushed back through my mind. Beau's one innocent question had brought up a thousand wounds. I couldn't tell him that I was engaged at nineteen or that the heartbreak from the engagement was still present three years later. He would think I was absolutely crazy. "Nope, nothing like that. A small heartbreak from my high school sweetheart," I lied. "But we all have that right?" I said casually.

"Oh yeah! You never love like your first love, and nothing ever hurts as bad as your first heartbreak," Beau said. "I think we've all had that."

PHEW! I thought. He didn't pick up on my lie. "Well, here we are! My apartment's up there," I said, pointing to the second floor, "so I guess this is goodnight."

"Goodnight, Rachel. I had a fantastic evening with you," he said, leaning in and delicately kissing my lips. The kiss felt genuine and refreshing.

We dated casually on and off again for the next two years, but I was never ready to commit. Commitment was all Beau wanted from me. I never called him my boyfriend; he never called me his girlfriend. We were open about the fact that we were dating other people. He asked me several times over those two years if I was ready to commit to our relationship.

"Don't you like things the way they are?" I always asked him. "They're easy and we're happy."

Every time I said that, I could see the hope dim a little more in Beau's eyes until what small piece of a relationship we had faded away, too.

You know when you meet someone great, but the timing in your lives is off? Well, for me, that was Beau. I always had fun with Beau, but I only ever let him see who I wanted him to see, never showcasing the scars of my past. I couldn't be authentic because with authenticity comes vulnerability, and vulnerability was out of the question. How could I even begin to share the heartbreak I held from the ex-fiancé and the community I had left behind in Indiana?

When I left Indiana, I didn't realize the emotional toll ending an engagement to an abusive partner or leaving a fundamentalist religion had had on me, until I started dating in Denver. I had learned everything I knew about relationships from John and fundamentalist religion, both of which now felt toxic to me. I knew I could never allow myself to enter a relationship like that again, so I denied myself the possibility of any truly intimate relationship. Looking back as part of my journaling homework, I saw that when I started dating in Denver, I was still in self-protection mode—survival mode. I thought, "If the man that proposed to me can abuse me and easily cheat on me, then how can I trust any man?" So I buried my emotions and placed an unbreakable lock on my heart.

About three years ago, after one very "Bad Date," I reached out to Beau for the first time in over a year, after our semblance of a relationship had fizzled. In our year apart, I experienced new traumas, and in response to this, I re-opened myself to therapy. During this time, one of the main growth points my therapist and I worked on was the power of forgiveness and the transformative power of vulnerability—the healing power that occurs when you are able to share your heart and your true self.

When I had to travel to Vail for the weekend for work and my company booked me in a two-bedroom condo, I immediately thought of inviting Beau to come with me. I wanted to see him and to apologize to him, so I invited him to come along. He happily agreed. During our first night in Vail, we sat on the couch in our condo rental and after a considerable amount of small talk, Beau looked at me and asked, "So Rach, don't get me wrong.

I'm happy to be here, but why now? Why did you want me to come with you after everything? I mean, we haven't talked in over a year."

I remember looking at him and feeling such guilt. I knew the pain I had caused him, and I wished so badly I could take it back, or that I could erase myself from his life. I felt the pain like it was my own. "Well . . . I guess I invited you here to apologize. I, um, I was in a really bad relationship before we met, and I didn't handle my life after it very well."

He stared at me blankly, almost in a daze.

"I just . . . I just feel terrible about the way I treated you. I wasn't ready to date, and I hurt you in an attempt to prove to myself I was ready. I'm just . . . so sorry." Shame rushed over me, like I was a little girl again running to the altar at church, confessing my sins to God.

Beau looked at me. His expression changed from shock to sympathy. He saw my heart and my heartbreak for the first time, and when he saw this, he wrapped me in his arms.

"I understand, Rach. It's okay. I forgive you."

After that night, we still never took our relationship past friendship. But in my hurt and vulnerability, I will never forget the compassion and kindness he showed me. Because of Beau, I began to trust again.

Throughout my entire life, I had longed for independence— for a voice. Now, finally, I had this freedom. I relished the independence I found in dating, unwilling to give up my newfound freedom for anyone. At the time, I didn't understand that there could be a balance between vulnerability and independence (two values never taught to me during my fundamentalist Christian upbringing), that without vulnerability, there cannot be true love, that in true love, there can still be independence.

Beau was the person that started me on the path to learn this lesson. When we were in Vail, and he held me in his arms, I felt the power and closeness that vulnerability creates between two people. I also felt the relief that comes along with vulnerability. In that moment, I felt like I removed a brick from the wall I had built around myself.

Just A Bad Date

In 2015, several months prior to my Vail weekend with Beau, I met Adam on Bumble, an online dating service. Adam had a dry, sarcastic sense of humor, which I loved. He was CEO of his own outdoor adventure company, which I loved even more. In addition to his humor and success, Adam had dark eyes and short light blonde hair. He was tall, athletic, and very handsome. After messaging me on Bumble for a week or so, Adam finally asked me over to his house for dinner. I quickly accepted his invitation. Adam seemed successful, funny, quick-witted, and handsome. I was ecstatic to finally meet him in person.

On a cold Thursday night in January, I went to Adam's house for dinner. I felt unsure about what to wear. It was a first date, but it was also a casual dinner at his house. I finally decided on black leggings and a Madewell flannel shirt—so I would look cute, but not like I was trying too hard. After fixing my curly hair and putting on some subtle makeup, I drove the five minutes over to Adam's condo.

When he welcomed me into his home, I immediately felt stunned. The condo was grand, with tall ceilings, large modern artwork on the reclaimed brick walls, and gorgeous mid-century modern furniture. The condo looked like an ad from West Elm come to life. I was also impressed by the way Adam looked in person. He was over six feet tall and had a great body. Immediately, I thought that I didn't belong here in this stunning condo with this beautiful man. I felt like he had made a mistake, and I was an unworthy imposter.

Adam took my coat and walked me through the small hallway to the large kitchen, which opened to the dining and living room. He had already begun cooking our dinner, so the house smelled like spices and Indian food.

"Can I offer you a glass of wine?" Adam asked with a smile.

"Sure! Thanks," I responded, as he poured me a glass of an expensive Cabernet Sauvignon. He handed me the glass, and I inhaled the aromas of peppercorn and raspberry. "So your place is really gorgeous!" I said in a tone that attempted to hide my surprise.

"Thanks! I bought it a few years ago when the market on this side of town had crashed. I'm pretty proud of the investment I made," he said, laughing. "Do you like to cook? I mean, would you rather watch me cook, or would you like to help, and we can cook together?"

I hesitated. I hated cooking. I would rather scrub bathrooms all day than cook a meal. I think this hate is partly because growing up in Evangelical Christianity, cooking was expected of women, especially good wives. I had cooked and helped my mom in the kitchen all my life until moving to Denver, when I realized that I didn't enjoy cooking at all.

Although I wanted to tell Adam, "No, thank you. I'll watch you cook," the words "Of course I can help you cook!" came tumbling out of my mouth before my mind had the time to contemplate them. It was as if I became a little girl again, back in my mom's kitchen, agreeing to help her cook out of female duty.

"Great!" Adam said, before pointing out what I could chop and mix for the recipe.

We laughed and played as we made dinner that evening. I almost felt like we could have been an ad for Green Chef or Blue Apron, cooking and candidly laughing in this West Elm kitchen. As we finished cooking, we plated our Indian chicken tikka masala, refreshed our wine glasses, and headed to his reclaimed wood dining table to eat. After sitting down, Adam immediately asked me, "What's your next dream that you'll achieve?"

Seeing my dumbfounded look at the depth of this question, he said, "Sorry if that caught you off guard. I want to get to know more of you than just the surface level. I'm kinda sick of going on these Bumble dates and leaving only knowing where the girl is from and what she does for work."

The expression on my face turned from dumbfounded to pleased. He didn't want me to hide. He wanted to see me. The other men I had been dating never pushed past my wall. To have Adam ask me this question at the start of our date felt refreshing and terrifying all at once. "I get it. Um, what's next . . . Well, I want to run a marathon. I've run six half marathons and the next thing I want to conquer is a full marathon."

"That's great!" he reassured me as our eyes met. "You can absolutely conquer that!"

"So, I guess I ask you a question now?" I said. "What is *your* next dream that you want to achieve?"

"Well, technically, you should ask me a new question," he said with a laugh, "but this will work. My next great achievement . . . um I want to hike Patagonia. I've been all over Central and South America for work, but never to Patagonia, so that's where I'll go next."

The night continued like this for the next three hours. Sitting at his kitchen table, we went back and forth with questions that led to deep conversations, then back to questions. We discussed poverty, socialism, feminism, work, family (his, not mine), and our love of the outdoors. Question by question, I felt more attracted to Adam—more in tune with him. When we had finished the bottle of Cab, I looked at the clock on the stove. It read 11:01 p.m.

"Oh shit! I didn't realize it was this late," I said, as I moved away from the table with my wine and plate. "I should go." I quickly texted my roommate, who I had instructed to call the police if she did not hear from me by 11:00 p.m., letting her know I was okay and on my way home.

Adam stood, too. "You don't have to go because it's late. We can keep talking."

"No, I um, better go. Thank you for having me. I had a wonderful night," I said, as I began to wash my dishes in the sink.

Adam came up behind me and kissed my neck. I immediately placed the wine glass down and turned around to kiss him. We kissed for a moment before I pulled away and walked to my coat. "Thank you again. Tonight was wonderful," I said, as I put on my coat and walked out the door.

The next morning at work, I couldn't stop smiling. Adam seemed amazing. The time we had spent together the night before was magical. With a giddy giggle, I told my coworkers how amazing my date had been and how badly I wanted to go out with Adam again. They all encouraged my excitement telling me that "he would definitely call me soon" and that "he sounds perfect."

Just like they said, he texted me within two days, asking if I was free for sushi the following Wednesday.

All week and weekend, I remember my excitement almost being too much to contain. Adam seemed like a perfect guy. With him, I had begun to let my guard down, which made me feel more connected to him than any other guy I had been dating. Finally, Wednesday night arrived! Adam picked me up around 7:00 p.m. in his silver Ford pickup truck. At five foot three, I grabbed the door handle and pulled myself up into his truck. Since Adam was taking me to a new, cool restaurant, I dressed up more for this second date, wearing black jeans, a white sweater, and black heeled booties.

"You made it!" he joked. "I forget how hard it is to get in this thing when you're short."

"Yeah. Good thing I'm athletic," I said with a laugh.

He took me to a posh sushi restaurant near his condo, and our conversation picked up like we had never left off. A few hours after we arrived at the sushi restaurant and our dinner was over, Adam looked at me and asked, "Would you like to come over for a glass of wine? Then I can take you home?"

We were still having a great conversation that I didn't want to end, so I nodded and said, "Sure. One glass of wine."

When we got to his condo, it was just as beautiful as I had remembered. Adam helped me take off my coat and began kissing my neck as he did so. The kisses were sweet and wanted. I looked at him and kissed his lips. The kiss felt better than the week before. Pulling back, I said, "Hey, just so we're on the same page. I'm not sleeping with anyone that I'm not in an exclusive relationship with." This was a rule I had made for myself a few months before in an attempt to eliminate the residual shame I still sometimes felt from having multiple partners.

After leaving the church, before my senior year at Indiana University, and experiencing freedom that came with sexual exploration, I went on somewhat of a sex "bender" for about three years. Having sex made me feel powerful, like I had complete control over my body and my pleasure (both of which John and the church had controlled until then). During this time, I always used condoms and was taking birth control, but more so out of secrecy than out of protection. I felt like as long as I used protection, no one would know about my "sex escapades" because there would be no STDs or pregnancy for proof. Sex became my secret escape where I found power and control, but after all these adventures, I decided that I wanted a life partner, not just a one-night stand. Even in my feelings of power and control over my life, the church still maintained some small power over me. I thought that in order to find a partner, I had to stop screwing on the first date so a man would want to be my partner. With this rule of "no sex until monogamy," I felt like a man would want me as his partner. *My value is my body. Sex outside of monogamy will leave me alone.*

He looked at me with lust in his eyes. "Are you sure I can't change your mind?" he said as he delicately ran his hand over my breast.

"Yes. I'm sorry, but I don't want to sleep with you yet."

He kissed me again before saying, "How about that glass of wine then?"

I stood against his white kitchen island as he poured us a glass of Pinot Noir. I breathed in the wine—cherries. I took my first sip. As soon as the glass left my mouth, he had grabbed it from my hands, placing both of our glasses on the island and pushing me against the fridge. He kissed me passionately, and I kissed him back. We stood there and kissed for a few minutes innocently, before I felt his hand pulling on the zipper of my jeans. He pressed all of his body weight into me, which made my moving away difficult, but I dipped under his armpit and moved to the kitchen sink across from the fridge, like a dance I learned in Cotillion.

I giggled innocently, hoping what I would say next would not make him angry. "Hey, I really like you, but I just want to keep this simple right now. I'm not ready for anything besides kissing."

"You're right. My bad, you're just irresistible," he said, with hunger in his eyes.

"Well, thank you," I said, as my hands picked up my wine glass. I moved to a stool on the opposite side of the island, unintentionally creating a barrier between us. "So, what are your plans for the rest of the week?" I asked, hoping we would be able to go back to a conversation.

"I'm going to go to the mountains on Saturday to take pictures for my portfolio." He moved to the side of the kitchen island where I was sitting and sat on the stool next to me. "I also hope I get to see you again." As he said this, his hand went to my thigh. I smiled. He knew how to flatter me.

"Well, maybe I'll let you see me again," I said playfully.

He leaned in to kiss me again. The kisses began gently, but after a moment or two, he slipped his hands behind my hips and pulled me on top of his lap. At this moment, something in me froze. I realized Adam was not listening to what I had said, and I didn't know how to get out of the situation. As I tried to politely pull away, he kept kissing me and pulling me closer. I moved my mouth from his and said again, "I really don't want this to go any further."

He looked at me with a smile, but it was not the smile that I had seen before. This smile was crooked and gave my body goose bumps. "You know you want me," he began. "Just admit it. Stop trying to play hard to get." At this point, he held me so tightly against his body that, when I used all my strength to pull away, I could only move a few inches from his face. Fear rushed through my body. "I do like you, and yes, of course, I'm attracted to you, but . . ."

He cut me off by pushing his face into mine. Then he moved his hands to my breasts. I took this opportunity to pull away and move backwards toward my stool. Before I could sit, he laced his hands behind my butt and picked me up—again pressing his face into mine and kissing me with unrequited kisses. Then he carried me to his bedroom across from the kitchen and placed me on his bed, using his body as a weight on top of me, so that I couldn't move. I lay frozen. *How had this escalated so quickly? I had said no, right? Right! I had said no multiple times. How do I get out of here? He is so much bigger than me, and he's on top of me.*

As my mind raced, Adam unzipped my pants and forced himself inside me. *What was happening? How do I make this stop? I said no. I know I said no.* I couldn't comprehend what was happening to my body. Tears began to silently stream down my face, colliding with his face, as he continued his forced kisses on my lips. Feeling my tears against his face, he moved his face from mine and looked down at me. I thought when he looked at me that he would see my fear, immediately realize what he was doing, and withdraw. Instead, he looked at me with hunger and flipped my body over so he could fuck me from behind. I lay like a corpse with frozen tears until he finished.

As soon as he was done, he kissed the back of my head, almost as if to say, "Thank you for letting me use you without a fight." Then he went to the bathroom. I lay on my stomach on his bed, unable to move—frozen, with my legs spread and my pants hanging at my ankles. I heard him flush the toilet and knew I needed to pull my pants up before he came back into the room. I rolled onto my back, pulled my pants up, and zipped them before

I rolled onto my side on the far left corner of his bed, placing my body into a small ball. Adam opened the bathroom door and walked back into the bedroom. He sighed a satisfied sigh, which made my stomach turn.

"That was great! Thank you."

I didn't answer.

"Rachel? Are you awake?"

Fuck, he thinks I'm asleep, so I'll pretend to be asleep. I let out a fake snore. He climbed to the opposite side of the bed and fell asleep with space in between our bodies. I remained frozen for the next six hours, unable to move or make sense of any of my thoughts.

As soon as I saw the sun come up, I tried to slowly crawl out of bed without waking Adam, but he rolled over. "Do you want a ride home?"

Still unable to speak, I nodded and walked to the door. He dropped me off at my apartment a few minutes later. The drive was silent until we arrived at my door. He looked at me with a smile. "Last night was great. I can't wait to see you again."

I felt crazy. *Last night was "great?" How could someone who seems so nice force himself on me? I mean, did he force himself on me? I didn't say yes. Did I? No, I definitely said NO multiple times.* I looked into his eyes for the first time since the night before and said, "Um yeah, I'm . . . um . . . kinda busy for the next few weeks but . . . um . . . you can text me."

He texted me the following week: "My dick is hard thinking about our night together. When can I see you again?"

I never responded.

That night, I realized that, even though I was no longer in the Evangelical Christian purity movement, I still had intense, conflicting feelings about consent. Consent is not discussed at all in the purity movement because sex is only meant between a husband and a wife. If your husband wants sex, it is "God's will" that you give it to him. In this purity culture, sexuality is all or nothing. You are either a known virgin or a whore with no room for the concept of consent. In this tradition, women are taught that they are responsible for the actions of men—that our "clothes" or "seduction" causes men to fall into sin. Sexuality and sexual sin are our fault, even if a man forces himself upon a woman. As my youth pastor once told me, date rape or rape by someone you know "is a terrible act, BUT God will forgive a woman only if she promises to never let a man fall into that sin again. Men want sex, and if you do not adamantly fight them off, then it is your body and your seduction that causes this terrible act."

Based on these sexist ideas, women are not empowered to make their own decisions regarding sexuality, and we are most definitely not empowered to tell men "NO." Through my Evangelical Christian upbringing, I learned that women did not have the right to make decisions about when to have sex and when to refuse it, and I knew about rape. But that night, I didn't know how to handle what had just happened to me and how my body had been violated. Although I had left the church almost four years before, the mindset of quiet submission was somehow still at work inside me. Even with all the freedom I felt and all the self-work I had done to become my own person, this night felt like the strongest reminder that *that* girl—that young, silent, and submissive Christian girl—still, despite all my work, lived inside of me.

I'm Okay

The morning after Adam sexually assaulted me, I went to my usual morning workout class. I thought it might help me mentally shut down for an hour—I wanted one hour of numbness. As I walked into the gym, I saw my friend Holly leaving. She smiled at me, sweat from her workout still dripping from her temples.

"Hey! I was just about to text you. How was your date with that guy last night? He seems amazing and . . ." Before she could finish, I began crying. She put her arm around me. "Rach, what's wrong? What happened?"

Through my tears, I kept repeating the same phrase over and over again, "I said no. I know I said no."

She pulled me out of the path of people, to the side of the gym for privacy. "Rachel, what happened?" she asked in a controlled, serious tone.

"I told him I didn't want to have sex, but . . ." I began in between heavy, tear-filled breaths, ". . . it happened, and I didn't run or scream or stop it."

Holly responded as only she would. She's a problem solver through and through and always speaks her mind. "I think you should go talk to someone. I have a great therapist. Can I give you her information?"

I nodded and hugged her. She whispered in my ear, "I'm so sorry." We stood there together for a minute before she recommended that I go home and sleep, instead of going to work out. I had already missed the first five minutes of class, so I agreed and drove home.

After a long nap that afternoon, I woke up and emailed Holly's therapist, Kathleen. My email was short.

> *Hello Kathleen,*
>
> *My friend Holly recommended me to you. I used to see a therapist, but I haven't been since I was in college three years ago. I think it's time for me to come back. Do you have an appointment this week or next?*
>
> *Cheers,*
>
> *Rachel*

She responded within an hour, offering her availability for the following week. I scheduled an appointment for the following Tuesday. For the rest of the week, I tried to push everything to the back of my mind, but that only made my anxiety run higher. So I decided to call my sister, Sarah.

Sarah and her husband had recently moved to Colorado Springs to be closer to me. Although she had followed what Mom and Dad expected of us—going to a Bible college (Moody Bible Institute) and marrying at the young age of twenty-one—Sarah had removed herself from the type of Evangelical Christianity we grew up in. She still believed in God, but as she had explained to me many times, "If the God we grew up knowing is the real God, then I would choose hell one hundred times over. I just don't believe that the God we grew up knowing is the real God. I believe in a God who loves everyone no matter what and who knows women are powerful, badass goddesses." She had almost been kicked out of Moody Bible Institute several times for voicing her "liberal" interpretation of the Bible, so I guess you could say that my sister is a rebel Jesus Feminist. Marching to the beat of her own song has never been a problem for Sarah, and I have always envied this quality of hers.

I called her over the weekend and explained what happened.

"WHO IS THIS FUCKING PIECE OF SHIT?" she screamed after listening to my story. I could tell that her anger had been building since I began my story, but she had patiently listened, like a woman wise beyond her twenty-two years.

"Well, I met him on Bumble," I told her.

"I KNOW where you met him. But who the FUCK is he? You need to go to the police now," she said, with virtuous anger in her voice.

"I already thought about that, Sarah. I can't. It will be a 'he said, she said.' Plus, the police can look at our phones, see that we had been on a date that night, and that we had flirted all day. They won't believe me. I'm not going to put myself through more trauma or embarrassment. I don't have any bruises. I'm not beat up."

She paused and inhaled deeply. "I'm sorry. I shouldn't have told you what to do." Her voice was calm for the first time since she had answered the phone. "I wish you would go to the police, but this is your trauma, not mine. Can I drive up and spend the weekend with you? We can eat pizza and watch *When Harry Met Sally . . .* on repeat?"

I needed my sister, my best friend. "Yes. I would really love that."

"Great! I'll be there in an hour," she said, before clicking off the phone.

We spent all weekend together in my bed, ordering food, watching old rom-coms, and belting Broadway show tunes at the top of our lungs. When I broke down into hysterical crying several times, she held me and told me over and over again, "This is not your fault," until my tears dried, and we began our next movie.

On Tuesday night, I arrived at Kathleen's office. I wasn't sure what I would tell her, if I would just spill it all right away, or if I would hide some pieces of the event in fear that she would judge me. I sat in the small office waiting room for one or two minutes before the hallway door opened, and a tall woman entered the waiting room. She looked at me and with a kind smile said, "Rachel?"

"Yes," I said, as I shook her hand and followed her through the door to her office.

She wore square blue glasses and wide-legged gaucho pants. I guessed her age to be around forty-eight, but her mature demeanor made it difficult to tell.

"Please," she said, as she motioned to the couch.

The room was similar to Dr. Polis's office. There were large bookcases against both walls. They were filled with psychology, psychiatry, and self-help books. She sat in a gray chair as I took my place on the far corner of the tan couch. I grabbed the corner couch pillow and clutched it in my lap.

"Well, Rachel," she began, as she pushed her glasses up her nose. "I want to tell you that my sessions are $175 per hour, and I do not accept insurance. Will that work for you?"

Shit, I thought. $175 was a huge increase from my $25 sessions at the IU Health Center. In this moment, I realized, though, that I couldn't protect myself because I couldn't afford to hide pieces of my story from her.

"Yes. That works," I said, as I mentally calculated how much I would need to budget monthly.

"Great," she said. "So, let's start from the beginning. You said in your email that you had been to therapy, but you stopped. What made you want to come back?"

Here goes nothing, I thought. "Well, I had something bad happen to me last week. And my friend Holly, she comes here, but I know you can't tell me that you know her. She told me to come see you."

"Gotcha. So you said, 'something bad.' Do you mind providing a little more insight?" Kathleen leaned in with her yellow pad of paper and pencil.

I breathed deeply and clutched the pillow closer to my stomach. She took note of my physical changes and wrote something on her yellow pad. "Well, last week I had sex with a guy, but I didn't want to. I told him I didn't want to. I mean I think I did. No, I *know* I did."

She adjusted her pencil. "Rachel, I am so sorry that this happened to you. May I ask you a question?"

I nodded at her with pursed lips, trying to push down the tears welling up inside of me.

"Why do you think that you didn't say no? Why are you

doubting yourself?" she asked. I could tell by her voice that she believed me. Tears streamed down my face. "I don't know. I guess because I said no. I said no over and over again, but I didn't fight or scream, so . . . yeah . . ." I couldn't continue speaking because my tears had taken over my voice.

Her face filled with compassion. She handed me a tissue. "Rachel, have you heard of fight or flight?" I nodded. "Well, what about freeze?" she continued, as I stared at her perplexed. "Freeze is also a natural reaction, as natural as fight or flight, and, honestly, more common. Freeze kicks in when our body notices things that our mind cannot comprehend, the things that would make it dangerous for us to fight or flee. Does that make sense?"

I sat in the corner of the couch, thinking.

Kathleen saw me thinking. After waiting a few moments, she said, "So when our body knows that it will threaten our life to flee or fight, it is intuitive enough to know that freeze will save us."

I looked at her, tears still sliding down my wet cheeks. "So this wasn't my fault?"

"No. No, it was not," she said as she fought back her own tears. "Rachel, I'm so sorry that this man took advantage of you. You had nothing to do with what he did to you. It is not your fault."

My tears had softened, as my mind raced. *So, this wasn't my fault? I wasn't bad? I hadn't caused this?* "But what do I do about it?" What she said made sense in my mind, but I didn't understand how to rid myself of the shame I felt.

"Well you can press charges . . . "

I cut her off. "No. I'm not going to do that. We went on a con-sensual date, and the police will see the texts that show this. I don't want to be humiliated by a system that doesn't believe victims."

"Survivors," she said, correcting me before moving on. "I understand, and I support your decision. I can help you work through this. Would you like that?"

"Yes, I would."

Kathleen looked down at her notes. "May I ask you anoth-er question?"

"Sure."

"Have there been other times in your life where a partner has ignored your 'no'? Where maybe you have felt forced to perform sexually when you didn't want to?"

My body immediately shook. I felt like a piece of electricity had run through my bones. John, for all those years, John. I said no. He manipulated me until my "no" became my knees being bent in front of his dick again and again. My mind raced as I connected the dots of abuse, which I had been trying to bury for years.

"I . . . I . . . think so. I think this happened with my ex-fiancé, too." I continued, "No, I know this happened with my ex-fiancé, all the time, for years," I said, as my eyes looked into hers. But this time, my eyes were filled with anger, not tears. I hadn't broken up with him because I was unhappy. I broke up with him because he sexually abused me—manipulated me. My body knew to flee, even when my mind could not understand why. My body, my *being* protected me.

For the next hour, I slowly recounted my relationship with John. Kathleen listened without condemnation as I spoke freely and out loud for the first time about what John had done to me—how he had used me for his sexual gratification while demeaning me and breaking my self-worth. I felt like my trauma poured out of my mouth, like my body had been waiting for me to acknowledge what had happened, and now that I had, I could not control my vulnerability.

We ended the session, and Kathleen gave me homework. She asked me to keep a journal in which I would write down every time my sexual assault by Adam or relationship with John came to mind. As she explained the homework, she also said, "Rachel, I would like for you to start to reframe your language. What John did to you was sexual assault, and what Adam did to you was rape. There is no doubt about that." She let out a small sigh and paused before she continued. "There is freedom in our words. What happened to you was not your fault. When you call these traumas what they are, you will feel power over your trauma and begin to heal."

I saw Kathleen twice a month for the next year. Although I don't believe that you can forget or move past sexual abuse and rape trauma, I now *do* know that you can heal. You can become stronger. My own journaling about experiences like those with Beau, Adam, and John taught me this. Kathleen taught me this. I will never forget one session in particular where Kathleen really helped me to understand the healing power that I held within myself.

I was back on her couch, but this time I was not clutching the pillow in my lap. Instead, I leaned in and spoke through a trembling voice. Kathleen and I were discussing fear, particularly how fear debilitates you and crushes your ability to grow. "I understand that fear is not transformative, but how do I get this out of my mind?" I asked.

"You have to acknowledge what you are afraid of," she said, as she sat up straighter in her chair. "What fear is driving you?"

I thought for a moment before I began. "I guess fear that I will be alone? Fear that what John told me is true, that I 'will never find anyone.' Fear that I will never do anything with my life. That I will be unsuccessful . . . "

Before I continued, Kathleen cut me off. "Okay, Rachel. But so what? So what if those fears come true?"

I stared at her blankly. What did she mean? "Well, um, if they come true, then I fail."

"No, Rachel. What happens to you? Failure doesn't happen to you."

"Um, I don't know."

"Come on. You know. What will happen?" Her voice, normally calm and soothing, changed to a harsher tone, the type of voice a football coach uses when his players need to make the right play to win a big game.

"I don't know," I said with frustration. "I don't know what will happen if my fears come true."

"Yes, you do. You know! Rachel, what will happen? What has happened when your fears have come true before?" She was leaning in and staring fiercely into my eyes.

I thought and stared down at the ground until I quietly replied, "I have been OKAY."

"Say that one more time, but in an active way."

"If my fears come true, I will be okay." It clicked. "I WILL be okay," I said with certainty.

Kathleen smiled. "Yes, Rachel. You will be okay."

Feminism

Early on the morning of January 27, 2017, I marched in the first Women's March after President Trump was elected. The morning was chilly, so I wore a gray puffy coat over my "Nasty Women" shirt. I refused to zip up my coat, so I could proudly display the message on my T-shirt. Because of the surprising amount of traffic the march brought to Denver that morning, my friend Stefanie was late meeting me downtown. I waited for her outside the light rail stop.

I will never forget sitting outside that entire hour, watching in awe as parents, children, men, women, old and young piled into the streets with their signs and pink pussy cat hats. I watched with envy as mothers brought their daughters, and fathers gladly accompanied their wives and children. I felt envious because I wished I had had this experience as a child and because I knew this powerful movement was something I would never experience with my mom or dad, who had told me earlier that week all the reasons this march went against the "will of God."

Then, all of a sudden, a feeling of gratitude completely filled me and drowned out all my envy. The quiet inner voice of my heart reminded me all I had overcome to participate in this historic day: the misogynistic, oppressive religion I had left; my relationship with John; my church community. As I stared at the people passing by, soft tears of hope fell down my cheeks. I remembered being fourteen years old and sitting at the kitchen table at my aunt and uncle's house—the "kids' table" as Sarah, I, and my cousins used to call it. We were lucky enough to have a white Christmas that year, and the pure snow powder shone bright outside the large kitchen windows. As Sarah and I sat at the kid's table with our cousin, Greg, we all impatiently waited for the adults to leave the kitchen so we could change the kitchen TV from Fox News to *A Christmas Story.*

My parents and my aunt and uncle were gathered around the TV watching as the Fox News reporter detailed the evils of the "uprising feminist movement" and the ways everyone could protect their children from this activism, which was "sure to damage them." Sarah and I were somewhat paying attention to the news, as much as two young girls can to the news on Christmas, but mostly we were shoving Norwegian pancakes in our mouth, betting who could eat the most before we made ourselves sick. I remember watching Sarah finish her third or fourth pancake when, from behind us, my uncle said, "Girls." We turned to face him. He looked at us with a serious expression, gazing through his large, wire-rimmed glasses. "Please promise me one thing. Promise me that no matter what you become, you will never become feminists."

As I sat in downtown Denver and thought about my uncle's request, a woman in her early sixties came up and tapped my shoulder. She had a pink pussy cat hat that her light gray hair curled out from under. "It's powerful, isn't it," she said, removing her knit pink gloves and handing me a small tissue for my tears.

I took the tissue and wiped my cheeks. "Yes. It really is. I . . . I didn't know I would feel this overwhelmed . . . in a good way."

She smiled. "This your first march?" I looked at her and nodded. "Well, you can't march without a sign!" She handed me a large blank white poster, which had been hiding behind her pile of pre-made signs. Then she handed me a black marker. "Here you go, honey. Now, whatcha gonna write?"

I looked at her and smiled before I bent on the sidewalk and wrote, "Proud Feminist and Nasty Woman." I beamed as I handed her back the marker. "Thank you." She gave me a quick hug before walking down the street to the start of the march.

Stefanie met me shortly after my encounter with this woman. We hugged and began our walk a few blocks down to the start of the march. For the next two hours, we marched a little over a mile. The streets were overflowing with thousands more participants than expected, causing the march path throughout downtown Denver to move at a snail's pace, but neither of us noticed.

Although Stefanie and I usually talked to each other loudly for hours on end, we both marched those entire two hours with silence between us. I'm not sure why she didn't say anything, but I was quietly experiencing a flood of memories. The power and magnitude of the energy that morning felt breathtaking. Step by step, I remembered moments that flooded my entire being, not just my mind, causing me goose bumps and tears. I thought of my old lime-green-and-blue room in Albany, Georgia. I thought of that little red book—my instructions for living as a Godly woman that my mother gave me as a child. I also remembered the first time I read *The Purity Myth* and the dozens of other feminist literature that opened my eyes to female freedom.

I thought back to Linda, the church member my parents forced me to talk to, and the complete shame I felt when she convinced me that I had experienced an orgasm. I remembered the abuse and manipulation I had endured for years at the hands of John. I thought of John's engagement to me on the beach in Michigan and when, after our breakup, how I thought I would never feel that love for someone ever again. Then I thought of my first year living in Denver. I remembered the rape I had experienced at the hands of Adam. I recalled the complete love I felt for my body when I learned how to pleasure myself.

Memory by memory, I relived my history, my life. I felt the ache from these memories, but the pain was quickly overcome by the confidence I felt as I reminded myself of all the ways I had overcome my experiences, of all the times my voice was silenced, then all the times my voice had now been able to scream. I marched with hope, and I shouted with power as I remembered all I had overcome to stand there proudly and be okay.

Seven years earlier in 2011, when I left John and subsequently the church, there were a lot of things I still didn't understand about my past. I just knew I needed to follow the small voice of survival inside me telling me to leave. Looking back now, I realize I didn't understand the power that the indoctrination by the church held over me and my life, that the shame and guilt I felt for my body and my sexuality controlled my every thought and action and wasn't normal or healthy. I didn't understand that in leaving John, I left an abusive relationship or even that there were other forms of abuse outside of physical abuse. I didn't know how alone I would feel after leaving the church. How in quitting the church, I walked away from the only community I had known for my entire life. I didn't understand how awkward and scared I would feel as I began navigating my life to find new communities—new places to belong and be supported. But I think that out of all the things I didn't know, I really didn't realize the peace and freedom I would find by leaving.

For most of my life, I had been taught that freedom and peace could only be found in "God's will" or "God's perfect plan." When I left John and the church, I thought I would never find peace or freedom because I was not living in God's will—a chilling realization to accept at the age of twenty. I just believed I would always feel empty; I would never be whole or fulfilled outside of God. But even in this dismal, new system of belief, something inside of me—a small, inner voice of survival—saved my life.

As humans, our transformations are not always immediate and at top speed. Many times, personal revision takes years. Sometimes it takes small, minute choices or decisions, all based on what you want. Then one day you realize that you are no longer the same person as when you arrived. You realize that pieces of you that were once locked shut are now wide open. It is at this moment that you can look back on your journey with pride. You realize that you survived the moments that you never thought you could. And you realize that you can do it again.

Leaving Fundamentalist Christianity did not happen overnight. I did not wake up one morning and say, "I am done with religion." Leaving the church and unlearning the indoctrination the church instilled in me took several years. It took thousands of small decisions—small daily mindset shifts from my once held patriarchal beliefs about my body, my worth, and my voice. Through these small decisions and mindset shifts, I slowly found myself. I found a vulnerability and independence. I found my own voice. I found feminism.

Epilogue

Today, I still live in Colorado with my adopted dog, Daisy. I see my parents, who live in Portage, two to three times a year. Although I am no longer a "believer" or a "Christian," we do not discuss my current belief system. They know that I do not go to church and that I do not have a Bible in my house (they still have over twenty-five Bibles in their house). Our relationship is good, but also fragmented, because I can never truly be my whole self around my parents. When I'm with them, I must revert back to a fraction of who I am now to make them feel comfortable.

I think that for them, if we verbally acknowledged that I am no longer a member of the church, they would have to recognize that their daughter, who they love, will be spending eternity in hell. They would feel like they had failed as parents, and I would never wish that burden on them. Mom and Dad brought me up in the church because they believed the church would be the safest place for me. My parents raised me according to the rules dictated by the church and the church's indoctrination. Mom and Dad followed these rules with only the best intentions. I understand the powerful hold that the church has on the lives of their members. I do not blame my parents for this. I still hope that one day we will be able to speak openly about our beliefs, with no judgment or tears, but with an understanding rooted in love.

Sometimes I think about what my life would have looked like if I had continued living within what the church told me was "God's plan." What if I had married John and lived with his abuse daily? What if I were to raise my own children within the shame-based, misogynistic religion that I'd been raised in? Who would I have become? Who would they become? When I think of this rigidly religious life—the life I thought I had to live—I smile with joy and relief that I'm living a much different life today. I feel proud when I remember the strength I had when I decided to listen to myself and leave everything I knew to follow that small voice of survival in my heart.

The life I had been told as a young person would grant me "peace" and "freedom" was a lie. That life, the life called "God's plan," would have been a life of religious oppression and continual abuse. Ironically, the life I'm living outside the church, the life I was told would lead to pain and ultimately "hell," has actually led me to a life of independence, confidence, freedom, and peace.

ACKNOWLEDGMENTS

Writing this book has been a journey filled with working late nights and weekends and experiencing both tears and joy. I want to thank everyone who called me or texted me such supportive messages that let me know you believed in me. Your words are what brought my story to life.

I would like to especially thank Clare, Lynsey, and Hilary for your constant support from reading and re-reading early drafts to providing feedback until the end. You all have been catalysts to this publication.

Sarah, you are my best sister friend. Thank you for allowing me to share parts of your story in sharing my own.

Laura, thank you for believing in the power of my story and reminding me of this when I felt doubt. Thank you for teaching me how to write and making this book a reality.

About the Author

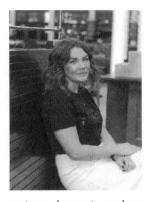

RACHEL OVERVOLL lives in Denver with her rescue dog, Daisy. Since leaving the church in her early twenties, Rachel graduated with a BS in Tourism Management from Indiana University. After college, she began a career in sales, enabling her to travel throughout the country.

Rachel has actively worked for women's rights, volunteering with various domestic and sexual violence organizations, including Project PAVE in Denver. She has also facilitated conversations around religion, feminism, body positivity, and privilege in her community.

Since leaving religion, Rachel has considered the open roads her church. She is a long-distance runner and has completed the Portland and Nashville marathons.

Contact with Rachel

RachelOvervoll

f Rachel.Overvoll